Palliative and End-of-Life Care

Editors

JAMES C. PACE
DOROTHY WHOLIHAN

NURSING CLINICS OF NORTH AMERICA

www.nursing.theclinics.com

Consulting Editor
STEPHEN D. KRAU

September 2016 • Volume 51 • Number 3

ELSEVIER

1600 John F. Kennedy Boulevard • Suite 1800 • Philadelphia, Pennsylvania, 19103-2899

http://www.theclinics.com

NURSING CLINICS OF NORTH AMERICA Volume 51, Number 3
September 2016 ISSN 0029-6465, ISBN-13: 978-0-323-46261-7

Editor: Kerry Holland
Developmental Editor: Casey Jackson

Nursing Clinics of North America (ISSN 0029-6465) is published quarterly by Elsevier Inc., 360 Park Avenue South, New York, NY 10010-1710. Months of issue are March, June, September, and December. Periodicals postage paid at New York, NY and additional mailing offices. Subscription price per year is, $155.00 (US individuals), $447.00 (US institutions), $275.00 (international individuals), $545.00 (international institutions), $220.00 (Canadian individuals), $545.00 (Canadian institutions), $100.00 (US students), and $135.00 (international students). To receive student/resident rate, orders must be accompanied by name of affiliated institution, date of term, and the signature of program/residency coordinator on institution letterhead. Orders will be billed at individual rate until proof of status is received. Foreign air speed delivery is included in all *Clinics* subscription prices. All prices are subject to change without notice. **POSTMASTER:** Send address changes to *Nursing Clinics*, Elsevier Health Sciences Division, Subscription Customer Service, 3251 Riverport Lane, Maryland Heights, MO 63043. **Customer Service: Telephone: 1-800-654-2452** (U.S. and Canada); **1-314-447-8871 (outside U.S. and Canada). Fax: 1-314-447-8029. E-mail: journalscustomerservice-usa@elsevier.com** (for print support) and **journalsonlinesupport-usa@elsevier.com** (for online support).

Nursing Clinics of North America is covered in *EMBASE/Excerpta Medica, MEDLINE/PubMed (Index Medicus), Social Sciences Citation Index, Current Contents, ASCA, Cumulative Index to Nursing, RNdex Top 100,* and Allied Health Literature and International Nursing Index (INI).

Printed in the United States of America.

Contributors

CONSULTING EDITOR

STEPHEN D. KRAU, PhD, RN, CNE
Associate Professor, Vanderbilt University School of Nursing, Nashville, Tennessee

EDITORS

DOROTHY WHOLIHAN, DNP, AGPCNP-BC, GNP-BC, ACHPN
Clinical Associate Professor and Director; Palliative Care Specialty Program, NYU Rory Meyers College of Nursing, New York, New York

JAMES C. PACE, PhD, MDiv, APRN, BC, FAANP, FAAN
Senior Associate Dean, Academic Programs and Clinical Professor of Nursing, NYU Rory Meyers College of Nursing, New York, New York

AUTHORS

TERRAH FOSTER AKARD, PhD, RN, PNP
Assistant Professor of Nursing; Co-Director, Pediatric Palliative Care Research Team, Vanderbilt University, Nashville, Tennessee

NINA BARRETT, NP, AGPCNP-BC, ACHPN
Palliative Care Nurse Practitioner, New York Presbyterian-Columbia University Medical Center, New York, New York

MARISSA N. BAUDINO, MEd
Vanderbilt University, Nashville, Tennessee

BARTON BOBB, MSN, FNP-BC, ACHPN
Palliative Care Nurse Practitioner, Thomas Palliative Care Services, Massey Cancer Center, Virginia Commonwealth University Health System, Richmond, Virginia

KATHLEEN BROGLIO, DNP, ANP-BC, ACHPN, CPE, FPCN
Section of Palliative Medicine, Dartmouth Hitchcock Medical Center, Lebanon, New Hampshire

COLLEEN FLEMING-DAMON, PhDc, APRN-BC, ACHPN, CT
Director of Education and Training, MJHS Institute for Innovation in Palliative Care, New York, New York; Doctoral Candidate, Adjunct Faculty, Adelphi University, Garden City, New York

MARY JO GILMER, PhD, MBA, RN-BC, FAAN
Professor of Nursing; Co-Director, Pediatric Palliative Care Research Team, Professor of Pediatrics, Vanderbilt University School of Nursing, Monroe Carell Jr Children's Hospital at Vanderbilt, Vanderbilt University, Nashville, Tennessee

ROSEMARY D. GORMAN, MSN, AGPCNP, ACHPN
Geriatric Health and Disease Management, RWJBarnabas Health, West Orange, New Jersey

MARY ELLEN HAISFIELD-WOLFE, PhD, RN, OCN
Division of Pulmonary and Critical Care Medicine, University of Maryland School of Medicine, Baltimore, Maryland

FLORENCE IYAMU, MS, FNP-BC, RN
University of Maryland School of Nursing, Baltimore, Maryland

KAREN SNOW KAISER, PhD, RN
Clinical Quality and Safety, University of Maryland Medical Center, Baltimore, Maryland

JANA LIPSON, RN, BA, BSN
Staff Nurse, Observation Unit, NYU Langone Medical Center, New York, New York

DEBORAH B. McGUIRE, PhD, RN, FAAN
Associate Dean for Research, Scholarship, and Innovation; Florence E. Elliott Professor, Virginia Commonwealth University School of Nursing, Richmond, Virginia

TYREE S. MOBLEY, BS, RN
Stroudsburg, Pennsylvania

JAMES C. PACE, PhD, MDiv, APRN, BC, FAANP, FAAN
Senior Associate Dean, Academic Programs and Clinical Professor of Nursing, NYU Rory Meyers College of Nursing, New York, New York

MARK RAMOS, RN, BSN
Staff Nurse, Medical-Surgical Unit, Northwell Lenox Hill Hospital, New York, New York

ANNA TIELSCH GODDARD, PhD, RN, CPNP-PC
Vanderbilt University, Nashville, Tennessee

CHARLES TILLEY, MS, ANP-BC, ACHPN, CWOCN
Palliative Care Consultant, International Advanced Practice Palliative Care Partners, LLC; Adjunct Faculty, New York University College of Nursing; Hospice Nurse Practitioner, VNSNY Hospice and Palliative Care, New York, New York

DONNA C. VICKERS, DNP, ANP-BC
Interventional Cardiology, Archbold Medical Group, Thomasville, Georgia

ANNE F. WALSH, ANP-BC, CWOCN, ACHPN
Visiting Nurse Service of New York, Hospice and Palliative Care, New York, New York

DOROTHY WHOLIHAN, DNP, AGPCNP-BC, GNP-BC, ACHPN
Clinical Associate Professor and Director; Palliative Care Specialty Program, NYU Rory Meyers College of Nursing, New York, New York

Contents

> Improved quality of life, care consistent with patient goals of care, and decreased health care spending are benefits of palliative care. Palliative care is appropriate for anyone with a serious illness. Advances in technology and pharmaceuticals have resulted in increasing numbers of seriously ill individuals, many with a high symptom burden. The numbers of individuals who could benefit from palliative care far outweighs the number of palliative care specialists. To integrate palliative care into primary care it is essential that resources are available to improve generalist palliative care skills, identify appropriate patients and refer complex patients to specialist palliative care providers.

> Animal-assisted therapy is an emerging complementary strategy with an increasing presence in the literature. Limited studies have been conducted with children, particularly those with life-threatening and life-limiting conditions. Although outcomes show promise in decreasing suffering of children receiving palliative care services, more work is needed to validate evidence to support implementation of animal-assisted therapy with this vulnerable population.

> Palliative care patients who have pain are often unable to self-report their pain, placing them at increased risk for underrecognized and undertreated pain. Use of appropriate pain assessment tools significantly enhances the likelihood of effective pain management and improved pain-related outcomes. This paper reviews selected tools and provides palliative care clinicians with a practical approach to selecting a pain assessment tool for noncommunicative adult patients.

Pain is a common occurrence in individuals with serious illnesses. Effective pain management can be complicated when the individual has a comorbid substance use disorder. Comprehensive pain assessment includes opioid risk screening to provide safe and effective pain management. An appropriate, safe treatment plan includes the use of "universal precautions" commonly used in managing chronic pain.

Palliative sedation has become a standard practice to treat refractory symptoms at end-of-life. Dyspnea and delirium are the two most commonly treated symptoms. The medications used in palliative sedation are usually benzodiazepines, barbiturates, antipsychotics, and/or anesthetics. Some ethical considerations remain, especially surrounding the use of palliative sedation in psychological distress and existential suffering.

An end-of-life vigil is the act of being with another toward death. A family vigil at end-of-life occurs when significant others gather by the bedside of dying individuals in the weeks, days, or hours prior to the death event. It is not unusual for nurses to be present, bear witness, and share in this human experience. This article reviews seminal and current research regarding the meaning and structure of the lived experience of vigil keeping for a dying family member, and translates research to inform nurses regarding family care during the transition at end-of-life.

Understanding the significance of rituals at the end-of-life enables health care professionals to offer meaningful and compassionate interventions that enhance quality of life and support those dying and those who grieve. Rituals contribute to the strength, capacity, and health of providers who cope with death events. Rituals help the living create continuing bonds with those dying, help with coping skills, and allow healthy growth through opportunities for naming, honoring, and memorializing. The display of respect and a nonjudgmental attitude create a space for support, trust, sharing of emotion, empowerment, and quality of care during end-of-life events.

Spiritual care is an integral part of multidimensional palliative care and a major domain of care identified in definitions and guidelines. Death bed phenomena include visions, dreams, hallucinations, and premortem energy surges, which can be deeply spiritual experiences. Death bed occurrences are often a source of consolation. However, they have been underrecognized. The last hours of life are sacred; as holistic, multidimensional practitioners, nurses should remain open to experiences not easily explained within a traditional medical model. As the most consistent caregivers, nurses assess, recognize, and validate such experiences to assist patients in finding meaning, comfort, and a peaceful end-of-life.

Nurses should be familiar with and equipped to address the challenges that arise when caring for lesbian, gay, bisexual, transgender, or queer-identified (LGBTQ) patients. LGBTQ individuals have increased rates of certain physical diseases and are at greater risk of suffering from stress-sensitive mental health issues. Negative social attitudes, widespread discrimination and stigma, physical and psychological victimization, and less social support with aging contribute to the complexity of care for these individuals. Open communication, welcoming and accepting attitudes and environments, and sensitivity to unique multidimensional issues improve care to LGBTQ patients with serious advanced illness. Nursing can reach this vulnerable minority and positively impact the quality of care.

Timely, holistic interventions aimed at easing the despair of patients with advanced cancer and malignant fungating wounds (MFWs) must incorporate patient and family goals of care in all aspects of decision-making. People with MFWs suffer from a devastating and often crippling symptom burden including disfigurement, pain, pruritus, malodor, exudates, and bleeding. These symptoms may lead to psychosocial and/or spiritual distress, isolation, and diminished quality of life. The complexity of caring for hospice patients with MFWs requires a pragmatic and holistic interdisciplinary approach guided by specialist-level palliative wound care. This article introduces a framework to assist clinicians in the assessment and management of terminally ill patients with MFWs.

NURSING CLINICS OF
NORTH AMERICA

THE CLINICS ARE AVAILABLE ONLINE!
Access your subscription at:
www.theclinics.com

Foreword

The Difference Between Palliative Care and End of Life Care: More than Semantics

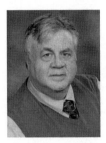

Stephen D. Krau, PhD, RN, CNE
Consulting Editor

Standards of end-of-life care and palliative care have been mutable over the last few decades. This is partially due to a lack of understanding about the differences between end-of-life care and palliative care. The differences are very explicit and important as decisions and plans are made for patients and their significant others. The concepts are similar but not the same.

Palliative does encompass end-of-life care, but it is so much more. Palliative care involves treatment of individuals who have a serious illness in which a cure or complete reversal of the disease and its process is no longer possible. It involves controlling symptoms that have either an insidious onset and progression or a rapid onset and progression. The purpose of palliative care is to assure the patient and those involved in his or her life experience optimal quality of life. This involves all dimensions of life, including symptom management, social, spiritual, and psychological needs. It involves care across the continuum of the patient's illness. A brief overview of the goals of palliative care is presented in **Box 1**.

End-of-life care is a portion of palliative care that is directed toward the care of persons who are nearing end of life. Although difficult to predict, end of life is care for individuals who are in the last year of life, and for legal and health care purposes, typically the last six months of life. End-of-life care is focused on maintaining quality of life while offering services for legal matters. A major component of end-of-life care is the focus on allowing patients to die with dignity.

When hospice care is considered, the boundaries among these three entities become more blurred. In essence, hospice care is similar to palliative care, but there are important differences. "Because more than 90 percent of hospice care is paid for through the Medicare hospice benefit, hospice patients must meet Medicare's

Nurs Clin N Am 51 (2016) ix–x
http://dx.doi.org/10.1016/j.cnur.2016.07.002
0029-6465/16/© 2016 Published by Elsevier Inc.

Box 1
The purposes of palliative care

To improve quality of life for the patient and his or her significant others

To provide relief from distressing symptoms and pain.

To support life and treat dying as part of a normal process

It combines spiritual and psychosocial aspects of care

It offers a support system to enhance active living during a disease process

Provides support for family coping during the disease process of the patient

It utilizes a team approach to care of the patient and his or her family

It does not hasten death, is focused on prolonging a life of quality.

Adapted from Marie Curie. Registered charity, England and Wales (207994), Scotland (SC038731). 2016. Available at: https://www.mariecurie.org.uk/help/terminal-illness/diagnosed/palliative-care-end-of-life-care. Accessed June 30, 2016.

---

eligibility requirements, which palliative care patients do not."[1] Similar to palliative care, the main objective of both is pain and symptom relief.

This issue of *Nursing Clinics of North America* focuses on interventions, modalities, and thought that can be and are considered with patients receiving palliative care, end-of-life care, and/or hospice care. In the current health care environment, it is not unusual to encounter patients in clinics, hospitals, or other settings that could benefit from palliative care. The focus and objectives of each transcends physical and geographical boundaries.

Stephen D. Krau, PhD, RN, CNE
Vanderbilt University School of Nursing
461 21st Avenue South
Nashville, TN 37240, USA

E-mail address:
Steve.krau@vanderbilt.edu

REFERENCE

1. VITAS Health Care organization. Available at: http://www.vitas.com/resources/palliative-care/palliative-care-vs-hospice-care. Accessed June 30, 2016.

Preface

Palliative and End-of-Life Care: Compassion, Care, Commitment, Communication, Communion

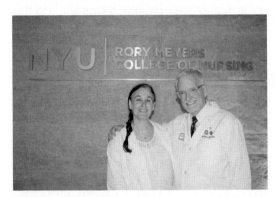

Dorothy Wholihan, DNP, AGPCNP-BC, GNP-BC, ACHPN
James C. Pace, PhD, MDiv, APRN, BC, FAANP, FAAN
Editors

We write this during National Nurses Week 2016, when we are reminded of how integral nurses are to the interdisciplinary team, and nowhere is this contribution more evident than in palliative care. Every nurse is a palliative care nurse. No nurse can escape the power and the promise of palliative care to look deeply into who our patients are and how we honor and support them. Nurses know that true person-centered care means assessing and addressing personal values, in addition to—and sometimes superseding—medical goals. As nurses, we often change the conversation, asking not, "What is the matter with you?," but instead, "What matters to you?"

We are honored to curate this very special issue of *Nursing Clinics of North America*. This issue offers visible signs of hope, courage, possibility, advocacy, and surprise. Our authors present novel and creative approaches to patient needs, thinking outside the box to address issues not often addressed and presenting unique approaches to meet them. Gilmer and her colleagues discuss the innovative use of animals to address the symptom needs of seriously ill children. Pace invites us to integrate use of ritual, as valued by the patient and family, to provide comfort to those who suffer and are bereaved. Our authors remind us that palliative care must spread to every setting and every person. Gorman helps us integrate palliative care practices into routine primary care encounters, while Barrett and Wholihan remind us of the unique needs of vulnerable populations like LGBTQ (lesbian, gay, bisexual, transgender, and queer [and/or questioning]) elders. In this issue, experts present us with strategies to address

Nurs Clin N Am 51 (2016) xi–xii
http://dx.doi.org/10.1016/j.cnur.2016.07.001
0029-6465/16/© 2016 Published by Elsevier Inc.

the most distressing and challenging symptoms we face: those areas of care where successful management seems sometimes out of reach. Tilley presents practical guidance for treating dreadful fungating wounds. McGuire and colleagues present the evidence for us to best understand and evaluate the pain experienced by those who cannot communicate, while Walsh and Broglio guide us the along the rocky path of pain management for substance users. Wholihan delves into end-of-life spiritual phenomenon not often brought out into the open, and Bobb presents an overview for the ethical use of sedation when the effective treatment of intractable symptoms eludes us. We thank each and every author for their passion, their spirit, and their commitment to what makes us human and tender and able to uphold and respect the dignity of life.

There is nothing more intimate, vulnerable, valuable, compassionate, spiritual, and set-apart than the work that is described in this issue. We invite you into every page. Take your time. We encourage you to be hopeful and to be proud of your work. Celebrate life and all that you do to make it truly worthwhile every day. You make a difference. Enjoy.

Dorothy Wholihan, DNP, AGPCNP-BC, GNP-BC, ACHPN
Palliative Care Specialty Program
NYU Rory Meyers College of Nursing
18 Commerce Street
New York, NY 10014, USA

James C. Pace, PhD, MDiv, APRN, BC, FAANP, FAAN
NYU Rory Meyers College of Nursing
433 First Avenue
New York, NY 10010, USA

E-mail addresses:
dw57@nyu.edu (D. Wholihan)
jcp12@nyu.edu (J.C. Pace)

Integrating Palliative Care into Primary Care

Rosemary D. Gorman, MSN, AGPCNP, ACHPN

KEYWORDS

- Primary care • Palliative care • Chronic disease • Symptom management
- Communication

KEY POINTS

- All nurses who provide consistent care are considered primary care providers (PCPs) and should be knowledgeable in the benefits of palliative care (PC) and adept at initiating PC.
- The focus of PC is the management of physical and psychological symptoms and spiritual distress in accordance with a patient's goals of care obtained through effective communication. The holistic care provided by nurses makes PC an integral part of practice.
- Improving access to PC for the nonhospitalized seriously ill would have a positive impact on the present health care system.
- Nurses have an ethical responsibility to advocate for end-of-life (EOL) care and serve as resources for patients and their families.
- PC is not the same as hospice; both are important in the management of serious disease.

PC is specialized care focused on the management of physical, psychosocial, and spiritual needs of patients and families experiencing serious illness. PC is about living and quality of life (QOL); it offers dignity and control. PC can continue until a patient approaches EOL and then transitions to hospice. PC can and should be instituted at any stage of illness and is appropriate concordantly with treatment to prolong life. Patients requiring PC can range from those requiring treatment of cancer to those with multiple chronic diseases. Even if full recovery is anticipated, PC can be appropriate. Currently, hospital-based PC specialists provide the majority of PC.

Because the focus of PC is on the management of physical and psychological symptoms and spiritual distress, PC may be appropriate multiple times throughout the trajectory of a serious illness. It is, therefore, essential that PCPs recognize the benefits of PC and become adept at initiating and providing generalist PC. In addition, PCPs need to be familiar with how and when to refer a patient to a specialist PC provider. Introducing PC in the emergency department (ED), the hospital, or the ICU

Disclosure Statement: The author has nothing to disclose.
Geriatric Health and Disease Management, RWJBarnabas Health, 101 Old Short Hills Road, West Orange, NJ 07052, USA
E-mail address: rosemarygorman312@gmail.com

is beneficial but often too late. Patients should not be subject to unmanaged symptoms or unnecessary care because it was never discussed. Inpatient PC should not be the gateway; PC should begin in primary care. PCPs and patients must be cognizant that PC is not synonymous with hospice care, and both are important in the management of serious disease.

PRIMARY CARE PROVIDERS

Primary care in the United States, as defined by the Institute of Medicine, is "the provision of integrated, accessible health care services by clinicians who are accountable for addressing a large majority of personal health care needs, developing a sustained partnership with patients, and practicing in the context of family and community."[1]

Primary care in the United States is the foundation of medical care and ideally the primary point of entry into the health care system. PCPs provide health promotion and preventive care, treat acute and chronic illness, and coordinate specialist care as needed. The goal for a PCP is patient-centered continuity of care that leads to long-standing relationships and effective communication. An established relationship with a PCP should ensure that changes in a patient's condition warrant evolving discussions about the specific impact of treatment and patient goals of care. Professionals caring for individuals who exhibit progression of illness are obligated to discuss prognosis and have a goals-of-care discussion with the development of a care plan reflective of these goals. This is an integral part of providing generalist PC. Research supports that EOL discussions are not associated with increased emotional distress. On the contrary, those who did not have EOL discussions had worse outcomes and their caregivers had increased emotional distress.[2,3] Lack of awareness regarding advance directives (ADs) was cited in a large study that reported only 25% of respondents having an AD.[4] Iterative discussions over multiple visits have shown to improve the completion of ADs.[5] An informed PCP considers the synergistic symptom burden, together with a patient's values and goals, and counsels patients accordingly, resulting in further discussions and shared decision making. Patients should be aware that treatment decisions left to a surrogate may cause significant burden. Additionally, often medical decisions regarding EOL made by a surrogate may be inconsistent with a patient's wishes.[2]

Primary care occurs in multiple settings, including offices, hospitals, outpatient clinics, rehabilitation facilities, long-term care facilities, assisted living facilities, and home care. This article specifically focuses on PCPs; however, all practitioners providing consistent ongoing care (ie, cardiology, nephrology, neurology, pulmonology, and oncology) should be knowledgeable and proficient in generalist PC and be cognizant of where and when to refer patients for specialist PC services.

Based on population growth, the aging population, and expanded health care coverage under the Affordable Care Act, the Association of American Medical Colleges predicts a shortfall of primary care physicians, ranging between 12,500 and 31,000, by 2025.[6] Although the number of primary care physicians is decreasing, the number of primary care trained nurse practitioners (NPs) is on the rise.[7]

The role of the NP is continually evolving, and NPs have the potential to fill the need for PCPs. NP care is safe, effective, timely, equitable, efficient, and patient centered. Literature supports NPs' contributions to high-value primary care.[8] Research by the Kaiser Commission on Medicaid and the Uninsured provides evidence that NPs are more likely to provide care to the uninsured and provide care in underserved areas and to the Medicaid population.[9] This is significant because an increased symptom burden is associated with poverty.[10] NPs' integration of PC is essential to the delivery of comprehensive, culturally competent primary care to diverse and vulnerable populations.

In addition to NPs, generalist nurses who provide consistent care to patients can be considered PCPs. Prime examples are long-term care nurses, nephrology nurses, outpatient oncology nurses, and home care nurses. These nurses see patients more frequently than primary care physicians and NPs and witness their patient's experience exacerbations, complications, and symptom burden. Ongoing trusting relationships are established over time; psychological and social aspects are included in ongoing care, all of which factor in to an individual's goals of care. Nurses also provide ongoing assessments of functional status, making dialogue concerning goals of care and EOL less intimidating and create an excellent opportunity to assist with advance care planning. Goals-of-care discussions held while a patient is conscious and competent not only add to patient satisfaction but add significantly to quality of care provided.[11]

The American Nurses Association (ANA) developed a formal position statement to reflect the code of ethics for nurses in regard to care at EOL. This article, entitled *Registered Nurses' Roles and Responsibilities in Providing Expert Care and Counseling at the End-of-Life*, can be accessed at the ANA Web site. It reads as follows:

The purpose of this position paper is to articulate the roles and responsibilities of registered nurses in providing expert end-of-life care and guidance to patients and families concerning treatment preferences and end-of-life decision making. It is meant to provide information to guide the nurse in vigilant advocacy for patients throughout their life span as they consider end-of-life choices.[12(p1)]

The ANA is clear on the nurse's role in supporting EOL care and its integration into primary care. The position paper further states,

Academic preparation and continuing education should prepare nurses to provide comprehensive and compassionate end-of-life care, so they can serve as advocates and resources for the patient and the patient's family. Expression of the patient's fullest autonomy in end-of-life decision making is best honored by addressing such questions in the primary care setting and throughout the life span, not only when a life-threatening condition arises. End-of-life patient counseling and education are "best practices" in all health care settings.[12(p2)]

Nurses caring for all patients with varying stages of chronic disease are uniquely qualified to facilitate advance care planning discussions.

BENEFITS OF PALLIATIVE CARE

Controlling symptoms is the cornerstone of PC. Individuals with chronic disease often experience high symptom burden. PC ensures care consistent with patient wishes established through effective communication and shared decision making. Increasing evidence shows that PC can improve QOL and symptom management, avoid unwanted procedures and transitions of care, eliminate unnecessary suffering, improve patient/family satisfaction, and decrease health care expenditures. Early PC can even improve survival is some cases.[13] PC also offers supportive care for family and caregivers, a crucial element in providing care during serious illness.[14]

Hospital PC programs in the United States have grown dramatically, enabling access in most large hospitals and academic medical centers to PC specialists. Disparities continue to exist, however, and are relative to geography, resources, hospital size, and ownership. The demand for PC specialists far outweighs the supply, and individuals with serious illness living in the community, nursing homes, and assisted living facilities have limited access to PC programs. This further reinforces the need for improved generalist skills. Creating access to PC for the nonhospitalized seriously ill who are not eligible for hospice care could be the single largest opportunity to improve the value in the present health care system.[15]

IDENTIFYING THE NEED FOR PALLIATIVE CARE

Technological advances in both the pharmaceutical and medical device industries have improved medical care and resulted in the increased survival of individuals with multiple chronic conditions. Dementia and diseases previously considered terminal, such as heart failure, chronic obstructive pulmonary disease, HIV, end-stage renal disease, and cancer, are now chronic long-term health conditions managed by PCPs and health care teams. Progressive chronic disease can have an uncertain illness trajectory, characterized by intermittent disease exacerbations, progressive decline in functional status, and associated high symptom burden. According to the Dartmouth Atlas of Health Care, 7 of 10 Americans die from chronic disease.[16] A dearth of evidence exists related to the management of multiple coexisting chronic conditions. This adds to the complexity of treatment and difficulty of prognostication. Geriatric syndromes, including frailty, falls, delirium, and incontinence, are common in older adults and can further lead to functional decline and an increased use of health care, including ED visits and hospitalization.[17] Individuals approaching EOL may experience frequent transitions of care undergoing treatment that has little benefit.

Estimates of life expectancy are influenced by the inclusion of functional status assessment over time.[18] This ongoing assessment alerts health care providers to a change in status and may influence appropriateness of interventions and treatment goals.[17] The annual Medicare wellness examination includes a functional assessment as well as a cognitive assessment.[19] Resources to assist with prognostication are found in **Table 1**.

Table 1
Prognostication resources

Resource	Source
The surprise question: Would you be surprised if this patient died in the next year?	The GSF Prognostic Indicator Guidance[20]
Palliative Prognostic Scale	Fast Fact #124[21]
Palliative Performance Scale	Fast Fact #125[22]
Mobile applications with prognostic indicators	Multidimensional Prognostic Index[23]— predicts short-term and long-term mortality in elderly subjects Qx Calculate[24]—helps determine prognosis in chronic disease
Prognosis Fast Facts (individual fast facts for chronic diseases)	Palliative Network of Wisconsin[25]
Global Deterioration Scale	GDS[26]

Abbreviation: GSF, gold standard framework.

GENERALIST OR SPECIALIST PALLIATIVE CARE
Generalist Palliative Care

Primary care practitioners as well as specialists who have not received specialty training in PC or hospice are referred to as generalist PC providers. The expectation is that all clinicians should be able to provide generalist PC.

Additionally, patients look to their primary provider for psychological support. It is unrealistic to rely on specialist PC providers to address all PC needs, because the numbers of seriously ill patients will continue to rise as baby boomers age. The generalist should also be knowledgeable in accessing community resources as well as providing caregiver support. Ideally, generalists provide ongoing PC and refer to PC specialists for the indications discussed later.

Specialist Palliative Care

Specialist PC is holistic care provided by a multidisciplinary team with specialty training/certification in PC. The team has expertise in the management of complex physical, psychological, social, and spiritual distress. The PC specialist may be necessary for refractory symptoms and complex family situations or when medical care is no longer beneficial. Most PC specialists are hospital based. Outpatient PC clinics are increasing in frequency. Home-based hospice companies use hospice and palliative-certified nurses and may also have a hospice-certified medical director and PC specialists.

Boxes 1 and **2** outline the skill set required for both generalist clinicians and specialist PC clinicians, according to Quill and Abernethy.[27]

CONTRIBUTIONS OF THE PALLIATIVE CARE GENERALIST
Physical and Psychological Symptoms

Decreasing symptom burden and improving QOL are the cornerstones of PC. Common symptom burdens associated with multimorbidity/complex disease include pain; anorexia/cachexia; anxiety; depression; fatigue; dyspnea; xerostomia; gastrointestinal symptoms, such as nausea, vomiting, and constipation; and sleep disturbances. These symptoms may occur alone or in multiple combinations and be related to a disease process or medications. A systematic assessment and good communication can lead to early identification of distressing symptoms, proper treatment and improved QOL.[14] Resources for the management of common symptoms are found in **Table 2**.

Communication Skills

Communication is the single most important element of generalist PC, because communication helps guide treatment and foster trust. Communication transcends all care settings. Patient-centered care requires that patients receive information to make health care decisions consistent with their needs, values, and preferences. Communication in PC should holistically address the physical, psychosocial, emotional, and spiritual needs of the patient. A patient's clear understanding of disease process, prognosis, and alternative treatments and its impact on overall QOL may result in early goals-of-care discussions affecting decisions about treatment,

---

Box 1
Primary palliative care skill set

Basic management of physical symptoms

Basic management of psychological symptoms

Basic discussions regarding diagnosis, prognosis, treatment goals, and code status

Adapted from Quill T, Abernethy AP. Generalist plus specialist palliative care- creating a more sustainable model. N Engl J Med 2013;368(13):1174.

> **Box 2**
> **Specialist palliative care skill set**
>
> Management of refractory pain and other symptoms
>
> Management of more complex depression, anxiety, grief, and existential distress
>
> Assistance with conflict resolution regarding goals or methods of treatment within family units, between staff and families, and among health care teams
>
> Assistance in addressing cases of near futility
>
> *Adapted from* Quill T, Abernethy AP. Generalist plus specialist palliative care- creating a more sustainable model. N Engl J Med 2013;368(13):1174.

interventions, and even rehospitalization.[33] Ultimately a goals-of-care discussion can lead to an AD, but this may be formulated over time and involve multiple discussions. Family involvement in these discussions has also shown to decrease nonbeneficial aggressive treatment.[34] When prognosis and full range-of-care options are not clearly discussed, patients may choose more aggressive care without fully understanding the effect of treatment on length and/or QOL. Schapira and colleagues[35] note that "Failure to prepare patients for death deprives them and their survivors of meaningful interaction that can never be replaced."

Communication skills are a primary component in specialist PC education, making palliative specialists skilled at active listening, resolving conflict, delivering bad news, and discussing issues of futility.[36] Generalists may benefit from additional formal academic or continuing education programs. Simulation is becoming increasingly popular as an effective teaching strategy to improve communication skills. Resources for practitioners to improve communication skills are found in **Table 3**.

Excellent communication includes up to date electronic medical record (EMR) documentation as well as the transfer of advance care planning documents across the continuum of care. EMR documentation should record the appointment of a health care proxy as well as the contact information and should reflect discussions of advance care planning, completion of documents, or changes in documents. The EMR should have a designated location for completed documents. Failure to communicate advance care planning documents when patients transition can result in unwanted aggressive treatment.

Community Resources

Although specialist PC is available in many acute care hospitals, patients who choose to remain or return home benefit greatly with referrals to appropriate community

Table 2
Symptom management resources

ELNEC	http://www.accn.nche.edu/elnec,[28]
Fast Facts (see individual symptoms)	http://mypcnow.org/#!fast-facts/c6xb,[29]
National Hospice and Palliative Care Organization	http://www.nhpco.org/education-online-learning/clinical topics,[30]
Relias Learning	https://reliaslearning.com/courses/library/advanced-palliative-care-30311,[31]
Center to Advance Palliative Care	https://www.capc.org/providers/courses/,[32]

Abbreviation: ELNEC, end-of-Life nursing education consortium.

Table 3 Communication resources	
Resource	**Source**
SPIKES protocol	6-Step protocol for breaking bad news[37]
Serious Illness Conversation Guide	SICG[38]
Delivering Bad News	Fast Fact #6 and #11[39]
Discussing DNR	Fast Fact #23[40]
Advance Care planning in Chronic Illness	Fast Fact #162[41]
Discussion points for providers	Sudore et al,[42] 2014 Spoelhof and Elliott,[43] 2014
Oncotalk	https://depts.washington.edu/oncotalk/,[44]
VitalTalk	http://vitaltalk.org,[45]

Abbreviation: DNR, do not resuscitate.

resources. Community resources include home care, day care facilities, and hospice as well as out-patient specialist PC providers.

Outpatient PC clinics are on the rise, allowing collaboration between the generalist and the specialist. Advantages of the outpatient PC clinic includes improving early access to PC; improved management of complex, challenging symptoms; and decreased utilization of health care resources, specifically the ED, contributing to both QOL and quality of death.[46,47]

It is important for the PCP to develop a relationship with a hospice agency. Some hospice agencies also provide community-based PC, which provides symptom management in combination with caregiver support and goals-of-care discussions earlier in the disease trajectory. The transition from PC to hospice at the terminal stage of illness can be facilitated by this ongoing relationship. The experienced clinicians in home-based PC/hospice can assist the generalist in complex symptom management, family support, and the identification of a patient that is hospice eligible.

SPECIALTY LOCATIONS
Pediatrics

Similar to the result of advances in technology, surgery, and pharmacotherapeutics for adults, children with complex health care needs and chronic illness are living longer. The prevalence of life-threatening conditions is increasing and approximately 8600 children are eligible for PC services daily.[48] Significant differences exist in the care of pediatric patients. The holistic care provided to a child/family, however, affected by a life-limiting illness can have a significant impact, the focus of PC being the child and family's QOL.[49] A policy statement released by the American Academy of Pediatrics in 2013 included a commitment that all clinicians should provide basic PC services and consult pediatric palliative and hospice care specialists in a timely manner.[50] Accessing pediatric PC services may be challenging depending on geography. Although there has been no recent formal survey of pediatric palliative services, the 2013 National Hospice and Palliative Care Organization national summary of hospice care indicated that only 14.1% of participating agencies have a designated pediatric PC staff.[47]

Liberman and colleagues[51] identified limited knowledge about ADs by the caregivers of children with chronic illness; however, the interest in creating an AD is great. Their interest should be a catalyst for ongoing communication with the PCP, optimally resulting in an AD and care consistent with goals. Unique to the pediatric population, under the Affordable Care Act, children covered under a state health insurance plan who are eligible for hospice care can continue to receive curative therapies while receiving hospice care.[47]

Home Care

Patients receiving home care services under Medicare are homebound. Increasing numbers of America's population are living with multiple chronic diseases and significant symptom burden. As disease progresses, functional status declines, care needs increase necessitating increased transitions of care, including EDs, hospitalizations, subacute rehabilitation facilities, and eventually home or long-term care. Curing and controlling disease inevitably must take a back seat, and comfort and QOL should become the priority.

Many patients with multimorbidity receive home care services after an acute exacerbation; home care nurses establish ongoing relationships with these patients and their families. The home care nurse's holistic approach of incorporation of physical, psychological, social, and functional status in the plan of care creates the perfect opportunity to address goals of care. The addition of PC to primary care in the home ensures adequate symptom management, avoids unnecessary transitions of care, and improves patient and caregiver satisfaction.[52]

Long-term Care

According to the Centers for Disease Control and Prevention, there are 15,700 nursing homes in the United States, housing 1.4 million residents.[53] Most residents of long-term care facilities have multiple chronic conditions and/or functional disabilities. Impaired cognition is a primary reason for long-term care and it is estimated that 70% of persons with advanced dementia die in nursing homes.[54] Most residents of long-term care remain there until their death. Pain is common in long-term care facilities and noted to be poorly treated for multiple reasons. Additional symptoms associated with chronic disease include dyspnea, neuropathy, weakness, depression, and feeding problems. Many long-term care residents would benefit from PC and hospice. Multiple challenges exist to providing PC in long-term care, including lack of knowledge among long-term care staff, frequent staff turnover, impaired cognition of residents, and lack of ADs on admission.[55]

Communication is paramount, because decision making and EOL care should be addressed with the family if a patient lacks capacity, ultimately resulting in an advance care plan. Interventions to Reduce Acute Care Transfers is a quality-improvement program specifically focused on nursing homes. It has an advance care planning communication guide for nursing homes that encourages all staff to participate in goals discussions.[56]

Hospice

Hospice is a type of PC that focuses on the final stage of disease. It provides interdisciplinary care to those with a terminal illness. Advantages of hospice care include improved QOL, avoidance of hospitalization, improved caregiver well-being, reduced health care costs, and improved patient family satisfaction.[57] Despite the growth of hospice care, it remains underutilized.[58] To qualify for hospice coverage under the Medicare hospice benefit, a probable prognosis of less than 6 months must be verified by 2 physicians and the recipient agrees to give up Medicare coverage for ongoing therapy or curative treatment of the terminal diagnosis.[59] Resources for hospice care and eligibility are found in **Table 4**.

Table 4 Hospice resources	
Medicare Hospice Benefit Part1: Eligibility and Treatment Plan	Fast Fact # 82[60]
Medicare Hospice Benefit Part 2: Places Of Care and Funding	Fast Fact #87[61]
Hospice in a Minute—provides types of service, admission guidelines, and hospice locator	Mobile app for IOS and Android[62]

REIMBURSEMENT

Recent changes to the Medicare system now support patient engagement in advance care planning with reimbursement for such discussions. The complexities and challenges of caring for patients with multimorbidity have also been recognized and reimbursement for non–face-to-face time is now covered under chronic care management. This allows PCPs to bill for close non–face-to-face follow-up. Specific information is available on the Centers for Medicare and Medicaid Services chronic care management Web site.[63]

Effective January 2016, Medicare Part B reimburses for discussions of beneficiary preferences for EOL care, otherwise known as advance care planning. The purpose of these conversations is to explore care choices if a patient were to become incapacitated or experience a life-limiting condition. Treatment choices, including resuscitation status, feeding tubes, and antibiotics, may be discussed. Advance care planning discussions do not need to result in an AD. Advance care planning is meant to be a series of discussions over time and should include disease progression and goals of care. The visit must be face-to face with the patient, family member(s), and/or surrogate. The Current Procedural Terminology codes are time based, with 99,497 to be billed for the first 30 minutes and 99,498 for each additional 30 minutes. Coding specifics can be accessed at MLN Matters number MM9271.[64] Verifying coverage for advance care planning is on an individual basis with commercial insurance carriers.

Chronic Care Management Services

In January 2015, Medicare began reimbursement for chronic care management services, a critical component of primary care, billable under Current Procedural Terminology code 99490 of the Medicare Physician Fee Schedule. This requires a minimum of 20 minutes of non–face-to face care coordination by clinical staff, directed by a physician or other health care provider (Advance Practice Nurse, Clinical Nurse Specialist, Physician Assistant) for Medicare beneficiaries with 2 or more chronic conditions.[63]

SUMMARY

PC is comprehensive and personalized care delivered together with ongoing treatment. The focus of care is on improving QOL for people facing serious illness. Emphasis is placed on pain and symptom management, communication and education about illness, medications, and what to expect as disease progresses. Ideally this process results in care consistent with a patient's goals of care and reduces both unnecessary suffering and unwanted treatment. Instituting PC early in an illness improves QOL and clear communication contributes to shared decision making between patient and provider.

Changes in functional status and repeat exacerbations indicate the need for ongoing communication and potential changes to goals of care. This is best done by the providers who have developed an ongoing relationship with the individual. Previously, PCPs responsible for holistic care of patients have lacked both the time and reimbursement for advance care planning discussions, but new Medicare guidelines allow practitioners to invest in this important communication. Integrating PC into primary care is essential to providing patient-centered care and can affirm life, promote QOL, and support patient and family.

REFERENCES

1. Primary care workforce facts and stats. Agency for healthcare research and quality website. Available at: http://www.ahrq.gov/research/findings/factsheets/primary/pcworkforce/index.html. Accessed January 11, 2016.
2. Kelly B, Rid A, Wendler D. Systematic review: individuals' goals for surrogate decision-making. J Am Geriatr Soc 2012;60:884–95.
3. Wright AA, Zhang B, Ray A, et al. Associations between end-of-life discussions, patient mental health, medical care near death, and caregiver bereavement adjustment. JAMA 2008;300(14):1665–73.
4. Rao JK, Anderson LA, Lin FC, et al. Completion of advance directives among U.S. consumers. Am J Prev Med 2014;46(1):65–70.
5. Ramsaroop SD, Reid C, Altman RD. Completing an advance directive in the primary care setting: what do we need for success. J Am Geriatr Soc 2007;55: 277–83.
6. The complexities of physician supply and demand: projections from 2013 to 2025. Association of American Medical Colleges (AAMC) website. Available at: https://www.aamc.org/download/426242/data/ihsreportdownload.pdf. Accessed January 13, 2016.
7. NP fact sheet. American Association of Nurse Practitioners website. Available at: https://www.aanp.org/all-about-nps/np-fact-sheet. Accessed January 11, 2016.
8. Naylor MD, Kurtzman ET. The role of nurse practitioners in reinventing primary care. Health Aff (Millwood) 2010;29(5):893–9.
9. The Henry J. Kaiser Family Foundation. Improving access to adult primary care in medicaid: exploring the potential role of nurse practitioners and physician assistants. Washington, DC: Kaiser Family Foundation website; 2011. Available at: https://kaiserfamilyfoundation.files.wordpress.com/2013/01/8167.pdf. Accessed February 16, 2016.
10. Beyea A, Fischer J, Schenck A, et al. Integrating palliative care information and hospice referral in Medicaid primary care. J Palliat Med 2013;16(4):376–82.
11. Ahia C, Blais CM. Primary palliative care for the general internist: integrating goals of care discussions into the outpatient setting. Ochsner J 2014;14: 704–11. Available at: www.ncbi.nlm.nih.gov/pmc/articles/pmc4295749/.
12. Position statement: registered nurses' roles and responsibilities in providing care and expert counseling at the end of life. 2010. Available at: http://www.nursingworld.org/MainMenuCategories/EthicsStandards/Ethics-Position-Statements/etpain14426.pdf. Accessed January 18, 2016.
13. Temel JS, Greer JA, Muzikansky A, et al. Early palliative care for patients with metastatic non-small-cell lung cancer. N Engl J Med 2010;363:733–42.
14. Kelley AS, Morrison RS. Palliative care for the seriously ill. N Engl J Med 2015; 373(8):747–54.
15. Dumanovsky T, Augustin R, Rogers M, et al. The growth of palliative care in U.S. Hospitals: a status report. J Palliat Med 2015;19(1):8–15.

16. The Dartmouth Institute. Care of chronic illness in last two years of life. The Dartmouth Atlas of Health Care website. Available at: http://dartmouthatlas.org/data/topic/topic.aspx?cat=1. Accessed January 8, 2016.

17. Leff B, Kao H, Ritchie C. How the principles of geriatric care can be used to improve care for Medicare patients. Journal of the American Society on Aging 2015;39(2):99–105. Available at: www.asaging.org. Accessed on January 8, 2016.

18. Keeler E, Guaralnik JM, Tian H, et al. The impact of functional status on life expectancy in older persons. J Gerontol A Biol Sci Med Sci 2010;65(7):727–33.

19. Medical Learning Network. The ABCs of the annual wellness visit (AWV). Washington, DC: Center for Medicare and Medicaid Services (CMS) website; 2015. Available at: https://www.cms.gov/Outreach-and-Education/Medicare-Learning-Network–MLN/MLNProducts/Downloads/AWV-Chart-ICN905706TextOnly.pdf. Accessed January 13, 2016.

20. Thomas K. The GSF prognostic indicator guidance. The gold standards framework website; 2011. Available at: www.goldstandardframework.org.uk. Accessed January 8, 2016.

21. Wilner LS, Arnold RM. The palliative prognostic score (PaP), fast facts and concepts #124. 2004. Available at: http://mypcnow.org/#!fast-facts/c6xb. Accessed February 16, 2016.

22. Wilner LS, Arnold R. The palliative performance scale (PPS); fast facts and concepts #125. 2004. Available at: http://mypcnow.org/#!fast-facts/c6xb. Accessed February 16, 2016.

23. De Petris MP. Multidimensional prognostic Index (iMPI). 2011. Version 1.01/IOS. [Mobile Application Software].

24. QxMD Software Inc. QxCalculate. Prognostic calculators. Updated November 8, 2015. Version 5.6/IOS. [Mobile Application Software].

25. Fast facts and concepts: prognosis. Available at: http://mypcnow.org/#!fast-facts/c6xb. Accessed February 11, 2016.

26. Reisberg B, Ferris SH, de Leon MJ, et al. The global deterioration scale for assessment of primary degenerative dementia. Am J Psychiatry 1982;139:1136–9. Available at: http://www.fhca.org/members/qi/clindamin/global.pdf.

27. Quill T, Abernethy AP. Generalist plus specialist palliative care- creating a more sustainable model. N Engl J Med 2013;368(13):1173–5.

28. End-of-Life Nursing Education Consortium (ELNEC). American Association of Colleges of Nursing website; 2016. Available at: www.accn.nche.edu/elnec. Accessed January 13, 2016.

29. Fast facts and concepts; symptoms/pain. Available at: http://mypcnow.org/#!fast-facts/c6xb. Accessed February 11, 2016.

30. National Hospice and Palliative Care Organization. Clinical topics. National Hospice and Palliative Care Organization website. Available at: http://www.nhpco.org/education-online-learning/clinical-topics. Accessed April 4, 2016.

31. Relias learning: learning management. Advanced palliative care. Relias learning LLC website. Available at: https://reliaslearning.com/courses/library/advanced-palliative-care-30311. Accessed April 4, 2016.

32. Center to advance palliative care. CME/CEU courses. CAPC website. Available at: https://www.capc.org/providers/courses/. Accessed April 4, 2016.

33. Chen CY, Thorsteinsdottir B, Cha SS, et al. Health care outcomes and advance care planning in older adults who receive home-based palliative care: A Pilot cohort study. J Palliat Med 2015;18(1):38–44.

34. Fawole OA, Dy SM, Wilson RF, et al. A systematic review of communication quality improvement interventions for patients with advanced serious illness. J Gen Intern Med 2012;28(4):570–7.

35. Schapira L, Moynihan J, Von Gunten CH, et al. Phase 1 versus palliative care: striking the right balance. J Clin Oncol 2009;27(2):307–8.

36. Pollak KI, Childers JW, Arnold RM. Applying motivational interviewing techniques to palliative care communication. J Palliat Med 2011;14(5):587–92.

37. Buckman RA. Breaking bad news: the S-P-I-K-E-S strategy. Community Oncol 2005;2(2):138–42. Available at: http://www.haifamed.org.il/pictures/files/%D7%91%D7%A9%D7%95%D7%A8%D7%95%D7%AA%20%D7%A7%D7%A9%D7%95%D7%AA.pdf. Accessed February 16, 2016.

38. Bernacki R, Hutchings M, Vick J, et al. Development of the serious illness care program: a randomized controlled trial of a palliative care communication intervention. BMJ Open 2015;5:e009032.

39. Ambuel B, Weissman DE. Fast facts and concepts #6 and #11; delivering bad news, parts 1 and 2. 2005. Available at: http://mypcnow.org/#!fast-facts/c6xb. Accessed February 16, 2016.

40. Von Guten CF, Weissman DE. Fast facts and concepts #23; discussing DNR orders-part 1. 2005. Available at: http://mypcnow.org/#!fast-facts/c6xb. Accessed February 16, 2016.

41. Davison S. Fast facts and concepts #162; advance care planning in chronic illness. 2006. Available at: http://mypcnow.org/#!fast-facts/c6xb. Accessed February 16, 2016.

42. Sudore RL, Knight SJ, McMahan RD, et al. A novel website to prepare diverse older adults for decision making and advance care planning: a Pilot Study. J Pain Symptom Manage 2014;47(4):674–86.

43. Spoelhof GD, Elliott B. Implementing advance directives in office practice. Am Fam Physician 2012;85(5):461–6.

44. Back A, Arnold R, Baile W, et al. ONCOTALK: improving oncologists' communication skills. Oncotalk website. Available at: https://www.depts.washington.edu/oncotalk. Accessed April 4, 2016.

45. VITALTALK. VItaltalk website. Available at: http://vitaltalk.org/clinicians. Accessed April 4, 2016.

46. Murphy A, Siebert K, Owens D, et al. Health care utilization by patients whose care is managed by a primary palliative care clinic. J Hosp Palliat Nurs 2013; 15(7):372–9.

47. Owens D, Eby K, Burson S, et al. Primary palliative care clinic pilot project demonstrates benefits of a nurse practitioner-directed clinic providing primary and palliative care. J Am Acad Nurse Pract 2012;24(1):52–8.

48. Friebert S, William C. NHPCO's facts and figures: pediatric palliative and hospice care in America. 2015. Available at: http://www.nhpco.org/sites/default/files/public/quality/Pediatric_Facts-Figures.pdf. Accessed February 16, 2016.

49. Crozier F, Hancock LE. Pediatric palliative care: beyond the end of life. Pediatr Nurs 2012;38(4):198–227.

50. American Academy of Pediatrics. Policy outlines core commitments of pediatric palliative, hospice care, vol. 34. AAP News; 2013. 11.

51. Liberman DB, Pham PK, Nager LA. Pediatric advance directives: parents' knowledge, experience, and preferences. Pediatrics 2014;134:e436–43.

52. Ornstein K, Wajnberg A, Kaye-Kauderer H, et al. Reduction in symptoms for homebound patients receiving home-based primary and palliative care. J Palliat Med 2013;16(9):1048–54.

53. Nursing Home Care. Center for disease control and prevention website. Available at: http://www.cdc.gov/nchs/faststats/nursing-home-care. Accessed January 11, 2016.
54. Ersek M, Carpenter JG. Geriatric palliative care in long term care settings with a focus on nursing homes. J Palliat Med 2013;16(10):1180–7.
55. Kaasalainen S, Ploeg J, McAiney C, et al. Role of the nurse practitioner in providing palliative care in long-term care homes. Int J Palliat Nurs 2013; 19(10):477–84.
56. Ouslander J. Advance care planning communication guide: overview. Boca Raton (FL): INTERACT website; 2014. Available at: http://www.interact2.net/docs/INTERACT%20Version%204.0%20Tools/INTERACT%20ACP%20Communication%20Guide%20Dec%2016%202014.pdf. Accessed February 16, 2016.
57. Kelley AS, Deb P, Du Q, et al. Hospice enrollment saves money for Medicare and improves care quality across a number of different lengths-of-stay. Health Aff (Millwood) 2013;32(3):552–61.
58. Aldridge Carlson MD, Barry CL, Cherlin EJ, et al. Hospices' enrollment policies may contribute to underuse of hospice care in the United States. Health Aff (Millwood) 2012;31(12):2690–8.
59. Aldridge Carlson MD, Twaddle ML. What are the eligibility criteria for hospice?. In: Goldstein NE, Morrison RS, editors. Evidence-based practice of palliative medicine. Philadelphia: Elsevier Saunders; 2013. p. 443–7.
60. Turner R, Rosielle DA. Fast facts and concepts # 82; Medicare hospice benefit-part 1: eligibility and treatment plan. 2007. Available at: http://mypcnow.org. Accessed February 16, 2016.
61. Turner R, Rosielle DA. Fast fact and concept #87: Medicare hospice benefit-part 11; places of care and funding. 2nd edition. 2007. Available at: http://mypcnow.org. Accessed February 16, 2016.
62. Georgia Regents University. Hospice in a minute. Version 1.0/Android (updated July 30, 2015), version 1.2/IOS (updated April 11, 2013. [Mobile Application Software].
63. Chronic care management services. Centers for Medicare and Medicaid Services (CMS) website; 2015. Available at: https://www.cms.gov/Outreach-and-Education/Medicare-learning-Network-MLN/MLNProducts/Downloads/ChronicCareManagement.pdf. Accessed January 13, 2016.
64. Medical Learning Home. Advance care planning (ACP) as an optional element of an annual wellness visit (AWV). Washington, DC: CMS website; 2015. Available at: htpps://www.cms.gov/Outreach-and-Education/Medicare-Learning-Network-MLN/MLNMattersArticles/Downloads/MM9271.pdf. Accessed February 16, 2016.

Animal-Assisted Therapy in Pediatric Palliative Care

Mary Jo Gilmer, PhD, MBA, RN-BC[a],*, Marissa N. Baudino, MEd[b],
Anna Tielsch Goddard, PhD, RN, CPNP-PC[b], Donna C. Vickers, DNP, ANP-BC[c],
Terrah Foster Akard, PhD, RN, PNP[d]

KEYWORDS

- Animal-assisted therapy • Pediatrics • Palliative care • Interventions • Suffering
- Evidence-based practice

KEY POINTS

- Animal-assisted therapy (AAT) may benefit children receiving palliative care through addressing physical, emotional, social, and spiritual issues.
- Rigorous longitudinal studies of AAT are needed as we strive to reduce the suffering of children with life-threatening conditions.
- Development, implementation, and evaluation of AAT evidence-based programs may be a powerful addition to conventional treatment.
- Benefits of ATT for adults include reduced anxiety, stress, depression, enhanced mood, increased socialization, and increased energy levels.
- Nonpharmacologic approaches to symptom management often decrease costs and noxious side effect.

INTRODUCTION

Children with life-threatening or life-limiting conditions and their parents, siblings, and friends often experience stress, loneliness, and anxiety. Families have identified stress, anxiety, pain, and separation as key contributors to low overall hospital experience ratings.[1–3] Although families generally rate doctors, nurses, and other health care providers high on patient satisfaction surveys, they often rate the overall experience of hospitalization low.[4,5] In the interest of improving families' experiences, a goal of the Institute of Medicine is for health care providers to focus on patient-centered,

The authors have no financial or conflict of interests to disclose.
[a] Pediatric Palliative Care Research Team, Vanderbilt University School of Nursing, Monroe Carell Jr Children's Hospital at Vanderbilt, Vanderbilt University, 417 Godchaux Hall, 461 21st Avenue South, Nashville, TN 37240, USA; [b] School of Nursing, Vanderbilt University, Nashville, TN, USA; [c] Interventional Cardiology, Archbold Medical Group, Thomasville, GA, USA; [d] Pediatric Palliative Care Research Team, Vanderbilt University, Nashville, TN, USA
* Corresponding author.
E-mail address: maryjo.gilmer@vanderbilt.edu

holistic care, which includes actions geared toward emotional support of children and their families to relieve fear, anxiety, and loneliness.[6]

Traditionally, anxiolytic therapies have been prescribed to assist in controlling anxiety in hospitalized children, but this therapy is often associated with high costs and harmful side effects, such as constipation and nausea.[7–9] Therefore, the advent of nonpharmacologic approaches to manage anxiety and loneliness through complementary therapies has drawn attention from both consumers and the medical community.[8,10] Approximately 40% of the US population uses complementary therapies, including meditation, deep-breathing exercises, yoga, massage, and diet-based therapies.[11] Complementary therapies used in conjunction with conventional treatment are intended to treat not only the physical manifestations of illness but also the emotional, social, and spiritual issues associated with disease, the very essence of palliative care.[8,12,13]

The human-animal bond continues to be a topic of exploration in research, philosophy, and psychology. Animal-assisted therapy (AAT) is considered to be a subset of complementary and alternative medicine because it adds to the treatment and affects the way a patient may experience symptoms.[14] The American Veterinary Medical Association (AVMA) estimates that 69.9 million US households own a pet dog, and 74.4 million own a pet cat.[15] Veterinary researchers have found that benefits to pet ownership include an increase in social interactions and attention, improvement in mood, and extended life expectancy.[16,17] Researchers have also found that being engaged with an animal decreases levels of the stress hormone cortisol while enhancing hormones such as oxytocin, dopamine, serotonin, and prolactin, which creates a sense of tranquility.[18]

BACKGROUND

A review of the literature through a systematic search of CINAHL, PubMed, Psych INFO, and Medline was the basis for the following synthesis of the use of AAT with children. Initial search terms included pet therapy and AAT, but more specific terms such as canine therapy and animal-assisted activities (AAA), and children, adolescents, and youth were then added to the search. Reference lists were used to conduct secondary searching for additional studies not found in the original review. The authors contacted Pet Partners and the AVMA for recommendations for additional information. Search results were limited to English, with no restrictions for dates, because the authors wished to include a historical perspective of AAT.

Therapeutic use of animals in association with symptom management has been practiced for thousands of years.[19] Florence Nightingale documented positive effects of animals and noted that small pets are often helpful companions for the sick.[20] As a social reformer who was proactive and innovative, she used animals as companions for both the disabled and the infirm. Nightingale noticed that animals assisted with the healing process of soldiers wounded during action in the Crimean War.[21] Soon afterwards, Sigmund Freud hypothesized that dogs had a "special sense" and believed that dogs could even judge the character of individuals. He owned 2 dogs and allowed one of them, Jo-Fi, to attend therapy sessions for the calming presence the dog brought to the session and the assessment of a patient's mental status.[22]

As a child psychologist in the 1960s, Dr Boris Levinson speculated that encouraging emotionally challenged children to take care of pets had calming and therapeutic effects on them.[23] As the author of *Pet Psychotherapy*, Levinson noted that including his dog, Jingles, in therapy sessions helped children to be less resistant and decreased their anxiety during interactions.[24] One previously mute child even spoke to Jingles, and Levinson theorized the dog was an extension of the therapy, even referring to the dog as a cotherapist.[25,26] Levinson often brought Jingles to sessions with other children and began to use the term "pet therapy" in 1964.[25]

Dr Samuel Corson followed Dr Levinson's work by using dogs to implement his biophysical research with in-patient psychiatric patients. As a professor of psychiatry and biophysics at Ohio State University, Corson housed the dogs in his research laboratory and studied the effects of stress on dogs. One instance often cited was of an adolescent with selective mutism who had been unresponsive to treatment. When a dog was brought to his room, the teen began speaking and was discharged shortly thereafter. Corson was called the "father of pet-assisted therapy" after conducting further systematic interventions with dogs and severely compromised patients, often with amazing success.[27] His articles documented positive social interactions, influenced by dogs who became companions in an inpatient psychiatric unit.[27,28] Some therapists labeled animals as "social lubricants" for patients, facilitating communication channels and becoming an easy topic for conversation.[26,29,30] Individuals who are somewhat withdrawn may participate in conversation more easily in the presence of a dog.[30]

Types of Animal-Assisted Therapy

Assistance in healing and health promotion may come from therapy or service animals, but clear distinctions exist between them (**Table 1**). Service animals are most often dogs and are trained for a specific purpose, which may include assisting with mobility or visual disabilities and are usually owned by the person for whom the service is provided. Companion animals are a subset of service animals and can be trained to detect health problems or disease in their owners, which may include preseizure activity, hypoglycemia, or even cancer through the sniffing of body fluids.[31] The actions of these animals are also legally defined and recognized by federal law.[30] Under the Americans with Disabilities Act, establishments are required to allow people with disabilities to bring their service animals onto premises where customers are allowed, such as restaurants, hotels, retail stores, taxicabs, and sports facilities.[32]

In contrast, therapy animals are not defined or regulated by the federal government. Therapy animals generally are not owned by the clients nor are the clients responsible for the animals' well-being. They are brought to the pet therapy session by the owners, who are called the "handlers" in these sessions. Therapy animals are also not subjected to the same extensive and somewhat rigorous training that service animals

Table 1 Differences between therapy dogs and service dogs	
Therapy Dogs	**Service Dogs**
Trained by handlers/owners to promote positive human-animal interactions, activity, and education	Trained with specific purpose
Visit various institutions (eg, hospitals, nursing homes, hospices)	Owned by person who needs help with disabilities
Provide emotional support, increase social interaction, and normalize health care environments	Help owner to attain safety and independence
Certified by licensing organization (eg, Pet Partners)	Legally defined and recognized

Data from Pet Partners, 2015.

endure.[30] However, both handlers and therapy animals are required to complete pre-requisite courses and tests offered through programs that provide certification to be licensed therapy animals (see **Table 1**).[33]

Defining Animal-Assisted Therapy

Kruger and colleagues[34] identified 12 different terms in the literature describing the phenomena of AAT and AAA as well as 20 different definitions of AAT. Such diversity and interchangeability in terminology and definitions have created confusion as to the exact context and purpose of AAT.[26] Therefore, recent AAT literature reveals efforts to narrow terminology and clarify pertinent differences between AAA programs versus AAT programs (**Table 2**).[26,29,35] Pet Partners is a national nonprofit agency that trains volunteers and evaluates animal handler teams for AAAs or AAT.[26,33] The organization, formerly known as the Delta Society, has trained thousands of handler/animal teams in companion animal and therapy animal programs.[33]

AAA is usually spontaneous, involves the patient's own pet, and does not include specific treatment goals.[26,33,35] On the other hand, AAT is delivered by specially trained professionals and volunteers with animals that meet specific criteria for the purpose of providing goal-directed cognitive and/or physical outcomes.[26,33,35] An additional, accepted term in the literature is animal-assisted intervention, which serves as an umbrella term for both AAA and AAT. A variety of different animals has been used for AAT, including felines, canines, rabbits, and horses.[26] However, a meta-analysis of AAT studies reported that the pattern of effect sizes and confidence intervals strongly suggests that canines have a greater chance of being effective compared with other animals.[29] Therefore, canines are the most common animal species used in AAT.[36]

Animal-Assisted Therapy with Adults

Because more work has been focused on AAT with adults, a review of those results helps to shed light on the use of AAT with children. Growing evidence shows that the animal-human bond may be used in a therapeutic manner with adults to provide

Table 2
Animal-assisted therapies versus animal-assisted activities

	Animal-Assisted Therapy	Animal-Assisted Activities
Definition	Often used with people who have physical, social, emotional, or cognitive needs	Often "Meet and Greet" Involve pets visiting people
Goals	Each session has specific treatment goals	No specific treatment goals
Activity	Specific treatment activities for each patient	Generally same activity with various patients
Charting	Required	Unnecessary
Visits	Appointments are scheduled	Spontaneous
Length of time	Predetermined	Spontaneous and may differ as desired
Exemplar	Goal: increase ambulation skills with a physical therapist Activity: child walks the dog short distance around facility	Child holds pet in a long-term care facility Dog performs trick in patient's room

Data from Pet Partners, 2015.

emotional support, increase social interaction, and make the hospital appear more homelike for patients.[21,35–45] Patient and staff acceptance of AAT in the inpatient setting has been favorable.[46] Nursing staff reports an openness and eagerness to include AAT in patient care.[47] In addition, nurses personally report decreased stress levels and improved morale when interacting with canines.[48,49]

Multiple benefits for adults in the inpatient setting include the reduction of anxiety, tension, and depressive symptoms.[50] In patients being treated for psychiatric disorders, AAT is associated with improved mood and socialization as well as decreased anxiety and depression.[21,38,39,41,43,44,51] Hastings and colleagues[50] reported that AAT increases positive mood and encourages socialization among patients, their families, and staff on burn units. High-risk antepartum patients who required at least 3 days of hospitalization for bed rest had significantly lower ratings of anxiety and boredom following AAT.[42] Inpatients being treated for cancer-related illnesses who received AAT indicated less anxiety and depression than those who did not participate in AAT.[45,52] Cole and colleagues[53] found that participation in AAT resulted in lower anxiety ratings in patients hospitalized with heart failure. Additional positive attributes associated with AAT have been described in the literature. Physiologic improvements such as decreased cardiopulmonary pressures and neurohormone levels were noted in heart failure patients receiving AAT.[53] Abate and colleagues[54] also noted that patients with heart failure participating in AAT demonstrated an overall increased willingness to participate in ambulation therapy and were able to walk farther than patients who did not participate.

Animal-Assisted Therapy with Children

Very few rigorous studies have been completed examining the effects of AAT on children in health care settings. Of the existing published AAT literature, many of the studies have been in adult populations with pediatric reports highly anecdotal in nature. In experimental studies within the pediatric population, physiologic, psychological, and emotional benefits have been supported, but limitations in design and sampling mitigate the evidence (**Table 3**).

Nagengast and colleagues[55] examined the effects of a companion animal on physiologic arousal and behavioral distress in children (N = 23) from 3 to 6 years of age during a physical examination. This study was one of the first reported that assessed AAT in a medical setting in the pediatric population. Researchers used a within-subject, time-series design to examine the presence or absence of a companion animal on systolic, diastolic, mean arterial blood pressures, and heart rates as well as peripheral skin temperature. The Observation Scale of Behavioral Distress

Table 3 Examples of goals of animal-assisted therapy	
Category of Goals	**Examples**
Cognitive	Increased knowledge of concepts (eg, intravenous, port) Increased vocabulary (eg, pain, intervention)
Motivational	Improved willingness to be involved in group activities Improved interactions with others
Physical	Improved fine motor skills Improved mobility Improved balance
Psychological	Increased self-esteem, increased attention skills, reduced anxiety or stress

Data from Pet Partners, 2015.

(OSBD) was used to measure behavioral distress. A multivariate analysis of variance (ANOVA; $P = .05$) analyzed main effects and interaction effects on the physiologic variables. Statistically significant decreases in systolic blood pressure, mean arterial pressure, and heart rate occurred with a companion animal present. A one-way ANOVA examining the OSBD scores was also significantly different, indicating a difference in behavioral distress when the dog was present or absent from the room. This study is particularly important because it laid the groundwork for future research related to the effects of AAT with children in medical settings and hospitals.

Kaminski and colleagues[56] further examined how AAT can affect children who are inpatient at a hospital. The investigators evaluated the emotional and physical impacts of AAT when used with hospitalized children (N = 70) compared with child-life activities such as structured crafts, playing games, cards, and video games.[56] Participants were inpatient and hospitalized with several major diagnoses, including hematology/oncology (33%), cystic fibrosis (21%), medical (17%), trauma (9%), transplant (7%), diabetes (7%), and surgery (6%). Before either intervention, researchers interviewed children and their parents or caregivers about the child's mood with the Reynolds Child Depression Scale and self-reported pain rating. Salivary cortisol was collected before and immediately following the intervention to measure cortisol, which is associated with increased adrenocortical responses and stress. Heart rate and blood pressure were also measured to indicate levels of stress. The sessions were recorded so that researchers could review the session and rate the child's affect to the AAT.[56] This study found more positive perceived child mood with patients who received an AAT intervention. During the AAT interventions, patients displayed more positive affect compared with other child-life activities. Although not statistically significant, researchers also found that levels of salivary cortisol decreased after AAT. An unexpected finding was that heart rates were higher in the AAT group compared with the child-life group before and after the intervention. Researchers hypothesized that this could have been due to anticipatory excitement about getting to see the therapy dogs.[56] Overall, these findings suggest that AAT can have a positive emotional effect and can decrease stress levels when used in children who are hospitalized. A major weakness of this study is the procedure for taking salivary cortisol levels, which were measured immediately after the intervention. Salivary cortisol levels may take up to 20 minutes to adjust after a stressful experience. The researchers recognize this limitation and report those results may not be accurate. Self-reported and parental-reported data may have introduced participant bias and further influenced results.

A few studies focused on the effects of AAT on pain in children. A quasiexperimental study examined how AAT affected perceived pain levels in hospitalized children.[57] Participants included children aged 3 to 17 years in an acute care pediatric setting with an existing established AAT program. The participants were put into 2 groups based on when the dog was present and if the child was fearful or allergic to dogs: a group that received an AAT intervention (n = 18) and a group that received an intervention that consisted of quiet relaxation time (n = 39). Baseline pain levels using the FACES Pain Assessment Scale, blood pressure, pulse, and respiratory rate were measured before the intervention and then repeated after the intervention. Both groups participated for 15 to 20 minutes. Cross-tabulation tables and χ^2 showed similar findings at baseline between the 2 groups. Pain scores were lower after the test in the intervention group ($P = .008$), but blood pressure and pulse did not change significantly. Researchers found the pain reduction was 4 times greater in the children undergoing AAT as compared with those relaxing quietly. Limitations to this study include a small sample size and lack of true randomization. The study was also stopped prematurely (before meeting required sample size) because the trained dog (a 13-year-old Springer spaniel) died before the completion of the study. This study also did not explore the duration of pain relief for these children. Sobo and colleagues[58] conducted a descriptive pilot study that evaluated AAT and child pain perception. Researchers measured levels of physical pain and emotional distress levels in children (N = 25) aged 5 to 18 years of age who had surgery and experienced postoperative pain in a tertiary care children's hospital. A pre-post, mixed-methods design collected measurements before and after the AAT intervention. In addition, patients and parents were asked to explain what they enjoyed about visiting with a therapy dog. Although the study was a feasibility research intervention in nature, researchers recognize and warn when interpreting results that the study intentions were to establish feasibility of the methodology and explore AAT intervention viewpoints. Different qualitative themes were identified, including the dog providing "distraction" from pain, pleasure and happiness, entertainment, reminding the child of home, keeping the child 0company, calming, and easing pain. Researchers found pain levels significantly decreased after the AAT intervention ($P = .001$) but again acknowledge the study limitations in small size, scope, and data collection pilot feasibility. An important finding, though, is that AAT seems to distract children from pain-related cognition as well as result in pleasant emotions in children who like dogs (**Fig. 1**).

A quasiexperimental study by Tsai and colleagues[59] compared the effects of AAT to completing a puzzle with a research assistant in order to further explore how using AAT may affect physiologic and psychological stress in hospitalized children ages 7 to 17 years of age. Children (N = 15) with acute or chronic conditions who were admitted to pediatric units of a hospital received both interventions in 6- to 10-minute sessions over 2 consecutive days. AAT for this study was defined as petting, touching, and brushing the therapy dog. Blood pressure and heart rate were measured at baseline and after intervention. The Child Medical Fear Scale was used to measure fear related to medical procedures, and the State-Trait Anxiety Inventory for Children was used to measure levels of anxiety in children. Blood pressure and heart rate were measured a total of 18 times throughout the study: before, during, and after the AAT interventions. Statistical analysis using multivariate ANOVAs found decreased systolic blood pressure with AAT when compared with the alternate intervention. Anxiety and medical fear were not statistically significant after the AAT visit when compared with the alternate intervention either.

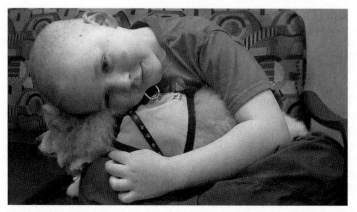

Fig. 1. Child receiving AAT. (*Courtesy of* Vanderbilt Medical Center, Nashville, TN.)

Calcaterra and colleagues[60] more recently published their findings from a randomized controlled pilot study with children (N = 40) between 3 and 17 years of age who were randomly assigned to either AAT (n = 20) or standard postoperative care (n = 20). Twenty-minute sessions with a therapy dog were conducted in postoperative patients, including orchidopexy, inguinal or umbilical hernia repair, circumcision, or varicocele surgeries. A complete electroencephalogram recording was obtained in the AAT patients and α activity was unchanged with no β activity recorded; however, after the entrance of the dog, diffuse βactivity was reported in all children receiving AAT, which researchers correlated with an increase in attention (βactivity). They also found a reduction in stress hormones as measured by repeated salivary cortisol. Major limitations to this study were again the small sample size.

LIMITATIONS

Several limitations in AAT published studies are recognized. Primarily, most of the literature with AAT and hospitalized children are either anecdotal or pilot studies. AAT is a very specialized complementary therapy requiring trained dogs or animals and their handlers. The intervention itself can sometimes be time-prohibiting, which further limits execution of studies with hospitalized patients. AAT can also last different amounts of times during visits as neither the animal nor the patient should be forced to interact with one another. Many of the reviewed studies recognize the lack of scientific data with a specific protocol for AAT. Many studies do not give specific details about the AAT and even fewer reported whether the dog was a companion animal or therapy dog. A wide variety of methods exist on how AAT can be implemented. Playing, petting, brushing, walking, and sitting with animals are all activities that are considered to be forms of AAT in some settings but may not meet formal criteria set forth by Pet Partners that is considered "therapy" versus animal "activities."

The published literature is often vague when reporting participant medical conditions, and few studies limit participation to patients with specific conditions. Many studies focused on pain reduction and required that the patient be reporting some level of pain in order to meet inclusion criteria. Broad inclusion criteria for research are not able to provide evidence on the effectiveness of AAT with certain subgroups within the pediatric population. None of the studies reviewed collected data over long periods of time and mainly focused on baseline and immediate postintervention measurements. This lack of longitudinal data fails to show whether the beneficial effects of AAT are sustained after the intervention.

Many of the studies reviewed relied on subjective self-report data. However, because pain is subjective in nature, findings continue to support a reduction in physical and emotional pain among children who participate in AAT.[58] Stress levels are also frequently measured by self-report instead of with stress cortisol levels, which are noninvasive and have been used successfully in prior research evaluating pediatric stress. Most of the participants in the AAT studies elected to participate in the intervention, indicating that participant bias may exist in the interventional research. AAT interventional studies are also limited in blinded methodology because patients will obviously know whether or not they received an intervention with an animal.

Most available literature did not give details or reports on the animals that were used in many of the interventions. Little to no information was provided on the dogs' well-being nor were any measurements reported. Braun and colleagues[57] reported that the canine used in their AAT study seemed to "take on the pain of the child," and the handler limited the number of intense sessions to no more than 3 a week. This same study reported that the therapy dog passed away during the therapeutic sessions, which stopped the study prematurely. Future research and interventions should consider the effect of AAT on the dogs as well as patients. Very few studies reported the number of dogs used in these studies nor how the handlers and their dogs were recruited for participation. Sobo and colleagues[58] proved a detailed description of their AAT intervention including descriptive information about Lizzy, the West Highland white terrier, and her handler, who performed the intervention. Information such as this is important to collect and report for methodology reporting as well as for future comparison research using canines in different health care settings.

Contraindications to Animal-Assisted Therapy

In some cases, children may not be interested in dogs or might even be allergic to certain animals.[30,61] Some children may have conditions that are agitated in the presence of certain animals, such as asthma or a pet-dander allergy.[62] Some children or families may actually be fearful of dogs or other animals. Therefore, individual assessment patients and possible contraindications to using an animal to facilitate therapy or treatment should be considered.[63] Most facilities have policies not allowing AAT visits with patients who are colonized with methicillin-resistant *Staphyloccocus aureus* (MRSA) or *Clostridium difficile*.[64] A state-of-the-science review by Urbanski and Lazenby[14] found that AAT should be avoided in high-risk patients that include

1. Severe allergies
2. Indwelling medical devices that cannot be secured or covered
3. Severe neutropenia (<500 neutrophils per microliter of blood), open wounds, or dermatitis that cannot be covered
4. Children with tuberculosis, salmonella, campylobacter, shigella, strep group A, MRSA, ringworm, and giardia
5. Children who have recent surgery or require sterile dressings, splenectomized children, and children with aggressive tendencies

Strong considerations should be given in using AAT in children who are immunocompromised and have moderate allergies.[14] A recent survey of top-ranked pediatric oncology hospitals found safety precautions differed across children's hospitals, but all had policies that required dogs receive yearly health examinations, be at least 1 year old, be on a leash or in a carrier, and that required children and handlers use hand sanitation after visits.[65]

PRACTICE IMPLICATIONS

Nurses often seek interventions to aid in physical symptom and stress reduction. Holistic nursing care involves facilitating healing and wellness beyond traditional medical treatment plans that often includes complementary therapies for the patient and family. Most AAT studies with pediatric patients report physical, psychological, and emotional benefits to the children.[57,58,66] Qualitative research and published anecdotal reports show animals may facilitate conversation, focus discussion, or break communication barriers.[21,58,66–69] Optimal pain management in pediatric patients continues to be of utmost interest to health care providers. Exploration of interventions for pain relief should remain a primary goal for pediatric nurse researchers.

AAT may not be beneficial to patients with

- Fear of animals
- Allergies to animals
- Asthma/respiratory problems

Researchers should take caution before requesting they participate in any AAT programs. Most facilities and hospitals have policies on pet visits and AAT programs that are implemented on the premises. Most settings require hand sanitizer use by the patient and the handler before and after visits, the placement of a clean towel or fresh linen on the bed or next to the bed where the animal will be used before the visit. Many AAT handlers discourage patients from feeding treats to the dog during visits, and the facility may also have a policy in this regard.[26,64] A canine consent form for the dog to visit while the child is hospitalized will also most likely be required.[58] Nurses and other clinicians caring for the patient should be familiar with infection control policies as they relate to animal visits at their facilities (**Fig. 2**).

CURRENT AND FUTURE RESEARCH

Further rigorous study of AAT, especially with children and teens, is indicated. Based on evidence from AAT in adults, AAT with children has the potential to decrease depression, anxiety, and pain, while improving activities of daily living and general well-being.[70] Studies are needed to explore the usefulness of AAT with a variety of diseases at various points along the illness trajectory with children in a variety of developmental stages. Additional or alternative outcomes, such as measures of self-esteem or long-term impact of AAT visits, could also be explored in different pediatric populations. Explorations of AAT using cats, rabbits, or even birds as a therapeutic milieu for children have yet to be explored and reported in the available published research.

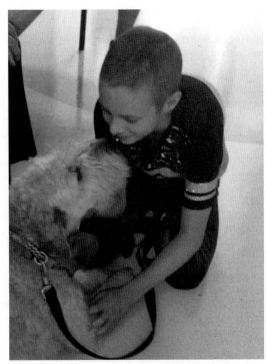

Fig. 2. Child interacting with dog during AAT. (*Courtesy of* Vanderbilt Medical Center, Nashville, TN.)

A lack of scientific data makes it difficult to define a specific protocol for AAT. Delivery of AAT currently differs from study to study, and specific details of the therapeutic interaction between the animal and child should be recognized. However, AAT may need to be altered or different based on the animal used. For example, some canines may have certain strengths, and their handlers may approach AAT slightly differently than others, and this limits the methodological rigor of a study that aims to standardize the therapeutic interaction and, therefore, fidelity of the intervention.

Few rigorous and peer-reviewed published studies show benefits to children's social, emotional, and cognitive development, possibly due to the aforementioned limitations in AAT research. The human-animal bond continues to be explored across multiple disciplines, such as veterinary medicine and clinical psychology, with a variety of variables under investigation. Dissemination of findings is critical to building the evidence for AAT as a complementary therapy and advancement of research in this field.

Finally, because of a lack of financial support for most experimental studies evaluating AAT, many studies are conducted with small convenience samples. No longitudinal studies to date have been published with AAT in pediatrics. Many of the published studies with animals have been conducted in the adult or geriatric population. Therefore, experimental studies with children examining potential outcomes are warranted as we strive to alleviate children's symptoms and treatment-associated stress.

Given the limitations of current research focusing on AAT with children, it is worthwhile to note a multisite multiyear innovative study that is currently underway designed to reduce the suffering of children newly diagnosed with cancer and their parents. The Canines and Childhood Cancer study that is led by American Humane Association and funded by Zoetis and the Human-Animal Bond Research Initiative is targeting ways to help these children who are 3 to 17 years of age. The study is currently being conducted at 5 children's hospital sites across the country, including Monroe Carell Jr Children's Hospital at Vanderbilt University, The University of California-Davis, Randall Children's Hospital, St. Joseph's Children's Hospital, and UMass Memorial Children's Medical Center, in partnership with Cummings School of Veterinary Medicine at Tufts University. The study goals include determining the feasibility and preliminary efficacy of AAT sessions on the outcomes of anxiety, stress, and health-related quality of life, using physiologic and psychological data. Preliminary results show a trend toward decreased pain and social challenges in children who received AAT.[71]

AAT holds considerable promise as an effective, holistic, complementary therapy to address physical and psychological symptoms in children with life-limiting or life-threatening conditions when using quality evidence to guide interventions. Potentially, through future development, implementation, and evaluation of more quality, evidence-based AAT programs, additional benefits of AAT will be realized, and widespread acceptance of AAT in pediatric palliative care as a powerful adjunct to conventional treatment will result.

REFERENCES

1. Cutshall SM, Fenske LL, Kelly RF, et al. Creation of a healing enhancement program at an academic medical center. Complement Ther Clin Pract 2007;13(4): 217–23.

2. Moser DK, Riegel B, McKinley S, et al. Impact of anxiety and perceived control on in-hospital complications after acute myocardial infarction. Psychosom Med 2007;69(1):10–6.

3. Muscara F, McCarthy MC, Woolf C, et al. Early psychological reactions in parents of children with a life threatening illness within a pediatric hospital setting. Eur Psychiatry 2015;30(5):555–61.
4. Coakley AB, Mahoney EK. Creating a therapeutic and healing environment with a pet therapy program. Complement Ther Clin Pract 2009;15(3):141–6.
5. Pelander T, Leino-Kilpi H, Katajisto J. The quality of paediatric nursing care: developing the Child Care Quality at Hospital instrument for children. J Adv Nurs 2009;65(2):443–53.
6. Institute of Medicine. Crossing the chasm: a new health care system for the 21st century. Washington, DC: National Academy Press; 2001.
7. Jiang W, Kuchibhatla M, Cuffe MS, et al. Prognostic value of anxiety and depression in patients with chronic heart failure. Circulation 2004;110(22):3452–6.
8. Ravindran AV, da Silva TL. Complementary and alternative therapies as add-on to pharmacotherapy for mood and anxiety disorders: a systematic review. J Affect Disord 2013;150(3):707–19.
9. Taniguchi S, Martins RM, Vogel C, et al. Initial palliative care drugs' side effect. Eur Psychiatry 2015;30(Suppl 1):1507.
10. Connor K, Miller J. Animal-assisted therapy: an in-depth look. Dimens Crit Care Nurs 2000;19(3):20–6.
11. Barnes PM, Powell-Griner E, McFann K, et al. Complementary and alternative medicine use among adults: United States, 2002. Adv Data 2004;(343):1–19.
12. Barnes PM, Bloom B, Nahin RL. Complementary and alternative medicine use among adults and children: United States, 2007. Natl Health Stat Report 2008;(12):1–23.
13. Tracy MF, Chlan L. Nonpharmacological interventions to manage common symptoms in patients receiving mechanical ventilation. Crit Care Nurse 2011;31(3): 19–28.
14. Urbanski BL, Lazenby M. Distress among hospitalized pediatric cancer patients modified by pet-therapy intervention to improve quality of life. J Pediatr Oncol Nurs 2012;29(5):272–82.
15. American Veterinary Medical Association. U.S. pet ownership and demographics sourcebook. 2012. Available at: https://www.avma.org/kb/resources/statistics/pages/market-research-statistics-us-pet-ownership-demographics-sourcebook.aspx. Accessed June 1, 2016.
16. Beetz A, Uvnas-Moberg K, Julius H, et al. Psychosocial and psychophysiological effects of human-animal interactions: the possible role of oxytocin. Front Psychol 2012;3:234.
17. O'Haire M. Companion animals and human health: benefits, challenges, and the road ahead. J Vet Behav 2010;5(5):226–34.
18. Creagan ET, Bauer BA, Thomley BS, et al. Animal-assisted therapy at Mayo Clinic: the time is now. Complement Ther Clin Pract 2015;21(2):101–4.
19. Stanley-Hermanns M, Miller J. Animal-assisted therapy. Am J Nurs 2002;102(10): 69–76.
20. Nightingale F. Notes on nursing: what it is, and what it is not. New York: D. Appleton and Company; 1898.
21. Chu CI, Liu CY, Sun CT, et al. The effect of animal-assisted activity on inpatients with schizophrenia. J Psychosoc Nurs Ment Health Serv 2009;47(12):42–8.
22. Fine AH. Handbook on animal-assisted therapy: theoretical foundations and guidelines for practice. 3rd edition. San Diego (CA): Elsevier Inc.; 2010.
23. Palley LS, O'Rourke PP, Niemi SM. Mainstreaming animal-assisted therapy. ILAR J 2010;51(3):199–207.

24. Levinson BM. Pet psychotherapy: use of household pets in the treatment of behavior disorder in childhood. Psychol Rep 1965;17(3):695–8.

25. Levinson BM. Pet-oriented child psychotherapy. Springfield (IL): Charles C. Thomas; 1969.

26. Fine AH. Handbook on animal-assisted therapy: theoretical foundations and guidelines for practice. 3rd Edition. Oxford (UK): Elsevier Science; 2010.

27. Corson SA, Corson EO, Gwynne PH, et al. Pet-facilitated psychotherapy in a hospital setting. Curr Psychiatr Ther 1975;15:277–86.

28. Corson SA, Arnold LE, Gwynne PH, et al. Pet dogs as nonverbal communication links in hospital psychiatry. Compr Psychiatry 1977;18(1):61–72.

29. Nimer J, Lundahl B. Animal-assisted therapy: a meta-analysis. Anthrozoos 2007; 20(3):225–38.

30. Rossetti J, King C. Use of animal-assisted therapy with psychiatric patients. J Psychosoc Nurs Ment Health Serv 2010;48(11):44–8.

31. Wells DL. Dogs as a diagnostic tool for ill health in humans. Altern Ther Health Med 2012;18(2):12–7.

32. U.S. Department of Justice. Commonly asked questions about service animals in places of business. 2008. Available at: http://www.ada.gov/archive/qasrvc.htm. Accessed June 1, 2016.

33. Pet Partners. Pet partners therapy animal program. Available at: https:// petpartners.org/volunteer/our-therapy-animal-program/. Accessed June 1, 2016.

34. Kruger K, Serpell J, Fine A. Animal-assisted interventions in mental health: definitions and theoretical foundations. Handbook on animal-assisted therapy: theoretical foundations and guidelines for practice, vol. 2. Oxford (UK): Elsevier; 2006. p. 21–38.

35. DeCourcey M, Russell AC, Keister KJ. Animal-assisted therapy: evaluation and implementation of a complementary therapy to improve the psychological and physiological health of critically ill patients. Dimens Crit Care Nurs 2010;29(5): 211–4.

36. Snipelisky D, Burton MC. Canine-assisted therapy in the inpatient setting. South Med J 2014;107(4):265–73.

37. Barak Y, Savorai O, Mavashev S, et al. Animal-assisted therapy for elderly schizophrenic patients: a one-year controlled trial. Am J Geriatr Psychiatry 2001;9(4): 439–42.

38. Barker SB, Dawson KS. The effects of animal-assisted therapy on anxiety ratings of hospitalized psychiatric patients. Psychiatr Serv 1998;49(6):797–801.

39. Barker SB, Pandurangi AK, Best AM. Effects of animal-assisted therapy on patients' anxiety, fear, and depression before ECT. J ECT 2003;19(1):38–44.

40. Berry A, Borgi M, Terranova L, et al. Developing effective animal-assisted intervention programs involving visiting dogs for institutionalized geriatric patients: a pilot study. Psychogeriatrics 2012;12(3):143–50.

41. Hoffmann AOM, Lee AH, Wertenauer F, et al. Dog-assisted intervention significantly reduces anxiety in hospitalized patients with major depression. Eur J Integr Med 2009;1(3):145–8.

42. Klemm P, Waddington C, Bradley E, et al. Unleashing animal-assisted therapy. Nursing 2010;40(10):12–3.

43. Lang UE, Jansen JB, Wertenauer F, et al. Reduced anxiety during dog assisted interviews in acute schizophrenic patients. Eur J Integr Med 2010;2(3):123–7.

44. Moretti F, De Ronchi D, Bernabei V, et al. Pet therapy in elderly patients with mental illness. Psychogeriatrics 2011;11(2):125–9.

45. Orlandi M, Trangeled K, Mambrini A, et al. Pet therapy effects on oncological day hospital patients undergoing chemotherapy treatment. Anticancer Res 2007; 27(6C):4301–3.

46. Nahm N, Lubin J, Lubin J, et al. Therapy dogs in the emergency department. West J Emerg Med 2012;13(4):363–5.

47. Tracy MF, Lindquist R, Watanuki S, et al. Nurse attitudes towards the use of complementary and alternative therapies in critical care. Heart Lung 2003;32(3): 197–209.

48. Carmack BJ, Fila D. Animal-assisted therapy: a nursing intervention. Nurs Manage 1989;20(5):96, 98, 100–1.

49. Rossetti J, DeFabiis S, Belpedio C. Behavioral health staff's perceptions of pet-assisted therapy: an exploratory study. J Psychosoc Nurs Ment Health Serv 2008;46(9):28–33.

50. Hastings T, Burris A, Hunt J, et al. Pet therapy: a healing solution. J Burn Care Res 2008;29(6):874–6.

51. Villalta-Gil V, Roca M, Gonzalez N, et al. Dog-assisted therapy in the treatment of chronic schizophrenia inpatients. Anthrozoös 2009;22(2):149–59.

52. Larson BR, Looker S, Herrera DM, et al. Cancer patients and their companion animals: results from a 309-patient survey on pet-related concerns and anxieties during chemotherapy. J Cancer Educ 2010;25(3):396–400.

53. Cole KM, Gawlinski A, Steers N, et al. Animal-assisted therapy in patients hospitalized with heart failure. Am J Crit Care 2007;16(6):575–85 [quiz: 586; discussion: 587–8].

54. Abate SV, Zucconi M, Boxer BA. Impact of canine-assisted ambulation on hospitalized chronic heart failure patients' ambulation outcomes and satisfaction: a pilot study. J Cardiovasc Nurs 2011;26(3):224–30.

55. Nagengast SL, Baun MM, Megel M, et al. The effects of the presence of a companion animal on physiological arousal and behavioral distress in children during a physical examination. J Pediatr Nurs 1997;12(6):323–30.

56. Kaminski M, Pellino T, Wish J. Play and pets: the physical and emotional impact of child-life and pet therapy on hospitalized children. Children's Health Care 2002; 31(4):321–35.

57. Braun C, Stangler T, Narveson J, et al. Animal-assisted therapy as a pain relief intervention for children. Complement Ther Clin Pract 2009;15(2):105–9.

58. Sobo EJ, Eng B, Kassity-Krich N. Canine visitation (pet) therapy: pilot data on decreases in child pain perception. J Holist Nurs 2006;24(1):51–7.

59. Tsai CC, Friedmann E, Thomas SA. The effect of animal-assisted therapy on stress responses in hospitalized children. Anthrozoös 2010;23(3):245–58.

60. Calcaterra V, Veggiotti P, Palestrini C, et al. Post-operative benefits of animal-assisted therapy in pediatric surgery: a randomised study. PloS One 2015; 10(6):e0125813.

61. Ernst LS. Animal-assisted therapy: paws with a cause. Nurs Manage 2013;44(3): 16–9 [quiz: 20].

62. Morrison ML. Health benefits of animal-assisted interventions. Complement Health Pract Rev 2007;12(1):51–62.

63. Novotny NL, Deibner J, Herrmann C. Animal-assisted therapy to promote ambulation in the hospital setting: potentially effective but is it feasible? J Nurs Educ Pract 2015;5(7):123.

64. Marcus DA. Complementary medicine in cancer care: adding a therapy dog to the team. Curr Pain Headache Rep 2012;16(4):289–91.

65. Chubak J, Hawkes R. Animal-assisted activities: results from a survey of top-ranked pediatric oncology hospitals. J Pediatr Oncol Nurs 2015. [Epub ahead of print].

66. Gagnon J, Bouchard F, Landry M, et al. Implementing a hospital-based animal therapy program for children with cancer: a descriptive study. Can Oncol Nurs J 2004;14(4):217–22.

67. Parish-Plass N. Animal-assisted therapy with children suffering from insecure attachment due to abuse and neglect: a method to lower the risk of intergenerational transmission of abuse? Clin Child Psychol Psychiatry 2008;13(1):7–30.

68. Silva K, Correia R, Lima M, et al. Can dogs prime autistic children for therapy? Evidence from a single case study. J Altern Complement Med 2011;17(7):655–9.

69. Borrego JL, Franco LR, Mediavilla MAP, et al. Animal-assisted interventions: review of current status and future challenges. Int J Psychol Psychol Ther 2014; 14(1):85–101.

70. Tielsch-Goddard A, Gilmer MJ. The role and impact of animals with pediatric patients. Pediatr Nurs 2015;41(2):65–71.

71. Gilmer MJ, Railey S, Akard T, et al. Are dogs really a child's best friend? European Association of Palliative Care International Conference, Copenhagen (Denmark), May 7–9, 2015.

Pain Assessment in Noncommunicative Adult Palliative Care Patients

Deborah B. McGuire, PhD, RN, FAAN[a],*, Karen Snow Kaiser, PhD, RN[b],
Mary Ellen Haisfield-Wolfe, PhD, RN, OCN[c],
Florence Iyamu, MS, FNP-BC, RN[d]

KEYWORDS

- Pain assessment • Noncommunicative or nonverbal patients • Palliative care

KEY POINTS

- Pain assessment of noncommunicative patients with a reliable and valid tool can provide consistency over time, enhance communication, and enable revision of the pain management plan.
- Vital signs may or may not provide a cue that pain is present and/or has been relieved.
- Preemptive pain assessment using a reliable and valid tool and intervention for pain-producing procedures may improve pain management and patient comfort.
- Some pain assessment tools are effective for assessing both pharmacologic and non-pharmacologic interventions.
- Incorporation of pain assessment tools into the electronic health record standardizes pain assessment and enables timely interventions and reassessment.

INTRODUCTION

The International Association for the Study of Pain's definition of pain—"An unpleasant sensory and emotional experience associated with actual or potential tissue damage, or described in terms of such damage"[1]—is widely accepted, but does not capture the complex multiplicity of physical, psychological, and spiritual dimensions encompassed in the experience of pain. Thus, pain is one of the most challenging clinical phenomena encountered by clinicians.

Disclosures: None.
[a] Virginia Commonwealth University School of Nursing, 1100 East Leigh Street, PO Box 980567, Richmond, VA 23298, USA; [b] Clinical Quality and Safety, University of Maryland Medical Center, 22 South Greene Street, Baltimore, MD 21201, USA; [c] Division of Pulmonary and Critical Care Medicine, University of Maryland School of Medicine, 22 South Greene Street, Baltimore, MD 21201, USA; [d] University of Maryland School of Nursing, 655 West Lombard Street, Baltimore, MD 21201, USA
* Corresponding author.
E-mail address: dbmcguire@vcu.edu

Nurs Clin N Am 51 (2016) 397–431
http://dx.doi.org/10.1016/j.cnur.2016.05.009
0029-6465/16/$ – see front matter © 2016 Elsevier Inc. All rights reserved.

nursing.theclinics.com

Although pain prevalence estimates vary by population and setting, it is not uncommon for 46% to 80% of individuals with chronic or terminal illnesses in hospital and hospice environments to have significant pain that causes both physical and psychological distress, interferes with activities of daily living, predisposes to development of adverse sequelae, impairs quality of life, and ultimately delays healing and recovery.[2,3] Prevalence estimates in palliative care populations that are not at the end of life are hard to find, and may be even higher than the figures cited. Palliative care patients who have pain at any point during their disease trajectory may be unable to self-report the presence, location, severity, or impact of their pain. They are considered at higher risk for underrecognized and undertreated pain, unnecessary suffering, or overtreated pain.[4,5] Recent evidence suggests that although nurses have beliefs about pain assessment and management in noncommunicative patients that reflect the American Society for Pain Management Nursing's prevailing clinical practice recommendations,[4] their knowledge and reported practices are not always commensurate with these recommendations.[6] The goal of palliative care in any clinical setting is to improve quality of life for patients who are facing life-threatening illness or injury by relieving pain, other symptoms, and psychosocial suffering, even when death is not the anticipated outcome. Although effective pain management is an important goal for all palliative care patients, it is especially important in noncommunicative patients.[5]

Pain management has been identified as a critical aspect of care by the Centers for Medicare and Medicaid Services.[7] From an ethical perspective, health care providers universally agree that all individuals have a right to the assessment and management of pain, a view also espoused by the Joint Commission.[8] Multiple position papers, clinical practice guidelines, and educational initiatives address pain management as a means to improve patient and family outcomes.[2,4,5,9,10]

Pain has long been considered an integrated "mind–body" experience in which the mind encompasses perception and interpretation of pain including affective, cognitive, and other responses, and the body encompasses pain pathways, central processing, and other phenomena that lead to perception and response. It is impossible to separate mind and body when considering the pain experience, hence the importance of self-report. Yet in noncommunicative individuals, the mind–body experience cannot be articulated through self-report. The International Association for the Study of Pain states that, "The inability to communicate verbally does not negate the possibility that an individual is experiencing pain and is in need of appropriate pain-relieving treatment"[1]; thus, clinicians need effective pain assessment approaches for this population.

The mind–body experience of pain can be conceptualized as having multiple dimensions (**Table 1**), each of which contributes to the overall experience of pain and has a role in pain assessment and management in all populations.[11] In those who cannot communicate, however, the physiologic and behavioral dimensions of pain are the most relevant, serving as a foundation for tools that use observable behaviors (eg, facial grimacing or restlessness) to assess pain, sometimes supplemented by physiologic indicators such as vital signs, which are used as cues for more in-depth assessment. Identifying the most appropriate behavior-based pain assessment tools for use in noncommunicative patients in any palliative care setting significantly enhances the likelihood of effective pain management and improved pain-related outcomes.[5] To date, few publications focus on development and use of pain behavior-based assessment tools in palliative care, other than in the end-of-life setting.[4]

The overall purpose of this paper is to provide palliative care clinicians with a useful approach to selecting and implementing a pain assessment tool for noncommunicative adult palliative care patients without dementia in various settings. Because pain

Table 1
Dimensions of pain and implications for assessment in self-reporting (SR) versus noncommunicative (NC) individuals

Type of population	Dimension					
	Physiologic	Sensory	Affective	Cognitive	Behavioral	Sociocultural
	Etiology, associated physiologic variables	How pain feels	How pain makes one feel	Perceptions, attitudes, beliefs	Pain-indicating or pain-relieving behaviors	Culture, meaning, beliefs, spirituality
SR	Cause of pain or syndrome Neurotransmitters Vital signs	Presence Severity Quality Duration	Mood Anxiety Irritability	Relief Coping Other	Sounds Movement Facial expression Muscle tension Guarding	Expression Management Other
NC	Vital signs may be cues	Does not apply	Does not apply	Does not apply	Behaviors indicating presence and possibly severity of pain	Does not apply

assessment in individuals with a diagnosis of dementia is complex and challenging, it is beyond the scope of this review and readers are referred to several comprehensive, evidence-based resources that focus exclusively on assessment of pain in the dementia patient.[4,12,13] The specific objectives of this paper are to (1) describe the psychometric and clinical properties of selected pain assessment tools for noncommunicative adult palliative care patients without dementia, (2) discuss key factors in selecting pain assessment tools for this population, and (3) present case studies from selected clinical palliative care settings to illustrate pain assessment in noncommunicative patients.

REVIEW OF SELECTED PAIN ASSESSMENT TOOLS

Pain assessment tools developed for use in various noncommunicative adult populations without dementia were selected for discussion if they met the following criteria: (1) published in English between 2000 and the present, (2) tested initially and/or subsequently in sample sizes with adequate justification for analyses, (3) demonstrated evidence of reliability and validity, with or without some evidence of clinical usefulness, and (4) tested in at least one clinical setting in which palliative care is delivered even if not acknowledged as such by the authors. Articles that described use of tools translated into non-English languages were excluded based on relevancy for North American readers, but English versions tested in other countries were included because there is no compelling evidence that patients' behavioral or physiologic responses to pain would be different. An iterative search of the PubMed and CINAHL databases yielded 7 tools that met these criteria, reviewed herein in alphabetical order. Articles detailing each tool's development and articles comparing it with other tools were analyzed on a number of parameters with the aid of methodologic and clinical usefulness resources and selected published systematic reviews.[14–18] Additional articles were included only if they provided other relevant insights. **Table 2** presents specific details on each tool's population/setting, psychometric research, and comments. **Table 3** presents information about clinical use of the tools, including administration time, training, clinical usefulness, scoring interpretation, and comments.

Behavioral Pain Scale

The Behavioral Pain Scale (BPS) was developed by Payen and colleagues[19] to assess pain in critically ill sedated and mechanical ventilated patients in a trauma and postoperative care unit. The BPS consists of 3 items using the following scoring system: (1) facial expressions (1 = relaxed, 2 = grimacing, 3 = lowering eyebrow, and 4 = closing eyelid); (2) movements of upper limbs (1 = no movement, 2 = partially bent, 3 = fully bent with flexion of finger, and 4 = permanently retracted); and (3) compliance with mechanical ventilation (1 = tolerating movement, 2 = coughing but tolerating ventilation for most of the time, 3 = fighting ventilator, and 4 = unable to control ventilation). The summed total score is unconventional because it ranges from 3 to 12. Subsequent research in other critically ill populations supported the validity, reliability, and usefulness of the BPS in assessing pain in critically ill, sedated, and primarily ventilated patients who could not self-report.[20–22] In addition, Ahlers and colleagues[23] examined the BPS in both conscious sedated patients and deeply sedated patients, demonstrating reliability and validity and suggesting that the BPS might serve as a "bridge" between an observational behavioral scale and a self-report pain assessment tool when patients have varying abilities to communicate pain. Recent comparisons of the BPS with other pain assessment tools in mostly noncommunicative intensive care unit patients generally found it valid, reliable,

Table 2
Pain assessment tools for patients who cannot provide self-report of pain: population, setting, reliability, and validity

Tool/Author	Population[a,b]/Setting	Reliability				Validity			FA	Comments
		IC	IR	T/RT	CNCT	PRED	DISC	CONV		
BPS[14,18–24]	• MV, sedated, with or without unconscious medical, surgical and traumatic head injury subjects • Some studies included MV subjects who could communicate at some time points • Single site studies in individual ICUs of various sizes from teaching hospitals or academic medical centers in France, Australia, Morocco, Netherlands, the Mid-Atlantic	A	AP	A	A	—	A	<A	A	• Overall, acceptable levels of IC, IR, T/RT, CNCT, DISC and construct validity (FA) to recommend use in practice with the critically ill patient • Further testing is recommended in noncritical care units and palliative care patients and settings • Validity and IR reliability may be inflated in some studies • Across studies, IR reliability seems to be high if raters have lots of experience using the BPS or if few raters are used • Sedation, iatrogenic or medically induced, may result in lower BPS scores • Ventilatory mode may affect scores • The upper end of the scale has not been tested
BPS-NI[28]	• Nonintubated/nontracheal medical/surgical ICU subjects with or without delirium • Medium sized ICU in a AMC in France	A	AP	—	—	—	X	—	X	• Preliminary evidence of IC, IR, DISC, and CNCT validity via EFA • Further testing is recommended in noncritical care units and palliative care patients and settings • IR reliability may be inflated • A comparison between the BPS and BPS-NI is recommended

(continued on next page)

Table 2
(continued)

Tool/Author	Population[a,b]/Setting	Reliability			Validity					Comments
		IC	IR	T/RT	CNCT	PRED	DISC	CONV	FA	
CNPI[29-31]	Predominantly Caucasian, hospitalized elderly female hip fracture subjects from 3 US Midwestern urban hospitals, undergoing surgery; of which 53 had on the average, moderate cognitive impairment from delirium or dementing illness; 73% were able to self-report	<A	M	—	<A	—	<A	—	—	• Evidence of moderate IR, close to acceptable IC and less than acceptable CNCT. No gold standard has been identified for patients who cannot self-report and may have influenced CNCT • Further psychometric testing is recommended in this, the critically ill, and in palliative care populations and settings • Limited IR testing suggests the CNPI: (a) may be overestimated, (b) needs further testing if only the movement related score is used, and (c) may be able to be used accurately by nurses. • IC was low, especially at rest and 3 behaviors were not seen in the study, suggesting the tool does not represent the constellation of pain behaviors seen in this population. Additional reliability and validity information related to dementia are reported elsewhere.

CPOT[27,37,41,43,46–48,54]   A

- Conscious/unconscious MV critically ill medical/surgical (including cardiac, trauma, and neurologic) subjects, including head trauma, some studies say no dementia.
- Small, medium, and large intensive care units in primarily university and teaching hospitals in Canada, and the eastern and central United States.

S to AP — X X X — — —

- Robust evidence of multiple types of reliability and validity in a tool that has also performed well in comparison with several other behavioral tools in critically ill MV patients; further work is suggested in palliative care patients across settings.
- The Faces Pain Thermometer, Verbal Descriptor scale and FLACC were used as gold standards, although these tools have not been identified as such.
- IR may be overestimated in some studies; however, numerous ICU nurses have used the CPOT with a large number of patients caring for a variety of patients, demonstrating it can be used reliably by nurses.
- Subsequent studies should clearly articulate which CPOT version is being used, the inclusion/exclusion criteria, and the population/setting.
- English and French version translation process should be clearly described and psychometric properties should be directly compared.
- Conscious patients may have higher scores than unconscious patients.

(continued on next page)

Table 2
(continued)

Tool/Author	Population^a,b/Setting	Reliability			Validity					Comments
		IC	IR	T/RT	CNCT	PRED	DISC	CONV	FA	
FLACC[46,53,54]	• Critically ill primarily medical subjects (including cardiac and neurologic) or immediate post cardiac surgery but also surgical, (including neurosurgical), with or without MV. • One small study (n <30) conducted in variety of critical care units from a medical center in the Great Lakes region contributed the most psychometric information; others were small single site studies (a cardiac postanesthesia care unit in a hospital in Northeast and a community hospital in the Mississippi Valley).	—	A	—	A	—	—	—	—	• Acceptable IR and CNCT, although small sample sizes and incomplete psychometric data (owing patient sample and study designs). • Further psychometric testing is recommended in this, the critically ill, and in palliative care populations and settings. • Although it has been purported to be the most frequently used tool in the critically ill, there is a lack of content validity (some items such as cry and consolability do not apply to adults). • Populations studied include some that are rarely included (neurologic, cardiac, and neurosurgical). • IR may vary by type of painful procedure and may be overstated.

| MOPAT[56-59] (McGuire, personal communication, 2016) | • Multiple studies using ethnically diverse medical and surgical subjects who were eligible to receive palliative care, many of whom were critically ill (including traumatic brain injury) or at end of life, who were experiencing acute procedural, uncontrolled, or episodic pain treated with a variety of nonpharmacologic and pharmacologic interventions.
• 22 intensive care and acute care units at an academic medical center in the mid-Atlantic and inpatient hospice units in the Southeast and Northeast. | A | X | — | — | — | X | — | X | • Demonstrates evidence of IC, IR and DISC and CNCT (FA) in ethnically diverse palliative care patients experiencing acute pain and receiving pharmacologic and non-pharmacologic interventions across multiple settings (acute care, including critical care, and inpatient hospice settings).
• Physiologic dimension has less than acceptable IC and needs additional exploration.
• IR varies by item; moderate levels of agreement for most items and for each dimension overall.
• The only tool to be assessed for reliability, validity, and clinical usefulness in palliative care populations experiencing uncontrolled or episodic pain.
• The only tool to be tested for reliability, validity, and clinical usefulness using a longitudinal design in a palliative care patient population.
• A comparison between the inpatient and hospice versions is recommended. |

(continued on next page)

Table 2
(continued)

Tool/Author	Population[a,b]/Setting	Reliability			Validity					Comments
		IC	IR	T/RT	CNCT	PRED	DISC	CONV	FA	
NCS[62–64]	• Subjects in an acute or chronic vegetative state or minimally conscious state experiencing experimental pain • Intensive care, neurology units, and long term care units in university hospitals, rehabilitation centers and long term facilities in Belgium and Italy	—	S to M	X	A	—	X	—	—	• Psychometric findings are based on experimental pain and demonstrate preliminary evidence of interrater reliability, test/retest reliability, as well as concurrent and discriminant validity; further psychometric testing is recommended in clinical palliative care populations. • The NCS did not discriminate between pain and no pain conditions, so it was modified by deleting the visual scale to create the revised NCS. • IR tested by minimal number of raters, none whom are identified as nurses, although it is a simple scale that could likely be used by a nurse; further testing is recommended.
Revised NCS[64,66]	• Subjects in an acute or chronic vegetative state or minimally conscious state • ICU and neurology units in a University Hospital (experimental pain and clinical pain), Neurorehabilitation Centers and Nursing Homes (experimental pain) in Belgium	—	—	—	—	—	X	—	—	• No reliability testing and minimal validity testing of the revised NCS English version, with 1 psychometric study using an experimental pain paradigm and 1 clinical study lending minimal evidence of discriminant validity; additional psychometric testing in a clinical population is recommended. • Demonstrates acceptable sensitivity and specificity in an experimental pain condition.

| NVPS[49,54,67,70] | • Critically ill subjects with trauma, surgery, and burn and open heart surgery
• Medium to large critical care units (1 mixed ICU and intermediate care) in academic medical centers and community hospitals in the Northeast, mid-Atlantic, Plains States, and Canada | <A to A | X, F | — | X to A | — | X | — | • Demonstrates preliminary evidence of reliability and validity; psychometric properties vary from study to study and may be related to population type.
• Has been compared with a variety of gold standards to assess concurrent validity, although a gold standard has not been identified for behavioral tools.
• IR is poor in some burn patient populations.
• The Physiologic 2 scale did not discriminate well between pain states and had the lowest correlations with other items on the scale, suggesting it should be modified. |

(continued on next page)

Table 2
(continued)

Tool/Author	Population[a,b]/Setting	Reliability			Validity					Comments
		IC	IR	T/RT	CNCT	PRED	DISC	CONV	FA	
NVPS-R[27,48,69-71]	• Critically ill medical, surgical, trauma, and neuro subjects (one-half of the latter could self-report) • Medium to large ICUs in academic medical centers in a Plains State, the Great Lakes region, and Canada • 1 LTC unit and 13 medical–surgical critical care units in 8 hospitals in the Midwest	A	N to S	—	<A	—	A	<M to M	—	• Demonstrates preliminary evidence of reliability and validity, but needs additional work as psychometric properties (may be population based such as ability to self-report or neurologic patients) and in comparisons with other well-established tools, it generally does not perform as well. • Cronbach's alpha is acceptable, except at rest, while IR is often lower than desired, even when compared with the NVPS. • Demonstrates discriminant validity; convergent validity results are often less than desired, although the gold standard selections are questionable. • Results are lower when used with patients who can self-report, confirming the importance of self-report.

Studies with conflicting levels of evidence: study designs were considered and the average level of evidence across studies was determined.

Studies using statistics other than those in **Table 2** of Gélinas et al[15] study design: statistical results were considered to assign a rating.

Abbreviations: AMC, academic medical centers; BPS, Behavioral Pain Scale; BPS-NI, Behavioral Pain Scale for nonintubated patients with delirium; CNCT, concurrent; CNPI, Checklist of Nonverbal Pain Indicators; CONV, convergent; CPOT, Critical Care Pain Observation Tool; DISC, discriminant; FA, exploratory factor analysis or principal components analysis; FLACC, Faces, Legs, Activity, Cry, Consolability; IC, internal consistency; ICU, intensive care unit; IR, interrater; LTC, long-term care; MOPAT, Multidimensional Observational Pain Assessment Tool; MV, mechanically ventilated; NCS, Nociceptive Coma Scale; NVPS, Nonverbal Pain Scale; NVPS-R, Revised Nonverbal Pain Scale; PRED, predictive; T/RT, test-retest.

Levels of evidence[15]: A, acceptable; AP, almost perfect; F, fair; M, moderate; S, slight; M, moderate; X, assessed.

[a] Unless otherwise specified, subjects were unable to self-report.

[b] All studies used adult subjects. In rare instances, studies also included 15- to 18-year-old subjects. Findings from these studies were included. If studies used a mixture of young pediatric subjects (<15 year olds) and adults, only adult findings are reported.

acceptable, and useful.[14,18,24] The BPS is supported by a large body of research and has been recommended for use in critical care settings for "monitoring pain in medical, postoperative, or trauma (except for brain injury) adult ICU patients who are unable to self-report and in whom motor function is intact and behaviors are observable."[25] It has also been paired with a pain protocol to improve pain outcomes.[26,27] The BPS was later revised to facilitate assessment of pain in nonintubated patients with delirium (BPS-NI), by replacing the compliance with mechanical ventilation item with vocalization (1 = no pain vocalization, 2 = moaning not frequent and not prolonged, 3 = moaning frequent or prolonged, 4 = howling or verbal complaint), although psychometric testing included patients without delirium and demonstrated preliminary evidence of reliability and validity.[28] A second study used both the BPS and the BPS-NI, treating them as 1 scale in the analysis.[27] However, there is no information about interpreting similarities or differences in scores between the BPS and BPS-NI. Neither of the BPS versions seems to have been tested in general palliative care patients with a variety of medical conditions, nor in intermediate care or noncritical care clinical settings, even though some patients, including the mechanically ventilated, are transferred to home or inpatient hospice units directly from a critical care unit. Both versions require additional exploration for use in nonintensive care palliative settings.

Checklist of Nonverbal Pain Indicators

The Checklist of Nonverbal Pain Indicators (CNPI) was modified from the University of Alabama Pain Behavior Scale as a measure of observable pain behaviors in patients greater than 65 years who had had surgery for a hip fracture and displayed varying levels of cognitive impairment from delirium or dementing illness.[29] The CNPI is a list of 6 pain-related behaviors (verbal vocalizations, nonverbal vocalizations, grimacing, bracing, rubbing, and restlessness) that are scored as present (1) or absent (0), both at rest and during movement (eg, transfer from bed to chair). Scores are summed for each condition (rest and movement) for a score ranging from 0 to 6, and then summed for a total score ranging from 0 to 12. Because the frequency of behaviors at rest was low, reliability and validity for the CNPI were reported only with movement. Comprehensive psychometric data were provided in a subsequent article,[30] showing that the CNPI had beginning evidence of reliability and validity and suggesting that it needed additional testing. For the cognitively impaired group, the CNPI was significantly correlated with the verbal descriptor scale at rest, so the developer suggested that the movement scale is more relevant.[31] Interrater reliability has only been reported for the tool as a whole. Interestingly, the cognitively impaired subjects displayed more nonverbal pain indicators than the nonimpaired subjects with movement. Because patients who can self-report pain demonstrate behaviors with movement at a less frequent rate, they may blunt pain behaviors with movement. Most tools, including the CNPI, have been tested using an acute pain paradigm; thus, their ability to determine underlying pain (eg, postoperative or persistent pain) is unknown. Some patients may need to be moved or subjected to pain-inducting procedures for them to be scored on the CNPI or other behavioral tools. The CNPI has not been tested in intubated, sedated patients in the intensive care unit, and its vocalization items may not be applicable in this population, thus restricting its use in the intensive care setting where there are numerous palliative care/end of life patients. Although there is little published evidence of additional psychometric evaluation of the CNPI, subsequent work conducted predominantly in nursing homes has catapulted the CNPI to some prominence as a tool for adults with dementia who are capable of varying levels of self-report.[32] However, the need for further psychometric and clinical evaluation has been highlighted in a study comparing the CNPI with the Pain Assessment in

Table 3
Pain assessment tools for patients who cannot provide self-report of pain: administration time, training, clinical usefulness, and score interpretation

Tool/Author	Administration Time	Training[a]	Clinical Usefulness[b]	Score Interpretation[c]	Comments
BPS[16,18–26]	• 1 min observation period • 2–5 min (includes scoring)	• In general, minimal descriptions and no consensus • Training, 15 d probation period, followed testing on a few patients • Standardized individual bedside training on 10 patients followed by interrater reliability testing • Pocket card (included BPS and graphic about contacting prescriber for BPS >5)	• Assessed as satisfaction • All agreed it took minimal time • 86% were satisfied with ease of use • 89% thought effective pain reactions during routine pain procedures had been assessed • 93% expected changes in pain assessment/relief owing to the BPS • 25% had concerns about complexity	• Lowest score (3) means no pain, but comparisons of BPS to Numerical Rating Scale and other scales implies a score of 3 may indicate pain, suggesting the BPS lacks sensitivity in detecting pain • Assumes a score of 12 is the maximal or highest pain, although no supporting statistical analyses • Several studies identified BPS scores >5 as indicating a need for intervention even though this score is higher than discriminant validity findings that suggest scores >4 indicate pain • Some items have been reported as ambiguous	• Recommend thorough training description and formal clinical usefulness analysis in a variety of settings and populations, including palliative care • Administration time is short • Unconventional scoring may be prone to misinterpretation • Needs testing to determine if scores relate to the various levels of pain and validate the score that indicates the need for treatment • Several studies used nurse raters, demonstrating the BPS is appropriate for nurses' use

BPS-NI[28]	Estimated to take 2–5 min to administer	• Standardized individual bedside training on 10 patients with follow-up interrater reliability testing • Training poster and pocket card included	—	• Lowest score is 3 (no pain) and 12 (most pain), but no confirmatory testing • Has not been tested to determine if it can discriminate between pain levels (none, mild, moderate, severe) or comparability to BPS	• Recommend a thorough training description and formal clinical usefulness analysis in a variety of settings and populations, including palliative care • Short administration time • Unconventional scoring may be prone to misinterpretation • Needs testing to determine a score that indicates treatment is needed and if the BPS-NI can discriminate between different pain levels • Clinical usefulness needs to be assessed by nurse clinicians
BPS-NI		• BPS and graphic about contacting prescriber for BPS-NI >5			
CNPI[29-31]	No information; appears easy to use	—	—	• Measures presence of pain, not severity • The lack of pain behaviors exhibited at rest suggests the CNPI rest scale is not sensitive and the tool developer suggests using only the movement scales • Has been integrated into an EHR in an inpatient hospice and acute care setting	• Thorough training description and formal clinical usefulness analysis in a variety of settings and populations, including palliative care are suggested • Administration time is short • Uses a 0–12 scale, different from frequently used self-report scales

(continued on next page)

Table 3
(continued)

Tool/Author	Administration Time	Training[a]	Clinical Usefulness[b]	Score Interpretation[c]	Comments
CPOT[2,7,37, 40–43,47,48,54]	15 s to (usually) 1 min observation time	• Training session of various lengths from undefined to <2 h that includes a description of the CPOT indicators and individual items, directions, scoring and documentation • With or without facial expression drawings; videotaped scenarios; ≥85%agreement; demonstration • Implementation study used educational sessions that included video demonstration of pain behaviors and instruction on applying the CPOT; physician and nurse champions; senior nurses who provided 1-on-1 bedside education and did compliance audits;	• All felt directions were clear and the CPOT was simple to understand • Overwhelming majority said it was quick to use, easy to complete, and the training time was sufficient • About three-quarters said they would recommend its routine use and that it was helpful for clinical practice • Slightly more than one-half said it influenced their pain assessment practice • Several nurses commented it offered a standardized, organized way to assess and communicate pain and that it encouraged sensitivity to nonverbal pain cues • A few individuals expressed concerns about the delay between training and use, the lack of specificity of some items, and that it could not be used with all ICU nonverbal patients	• Score range 0–8, with a different scale and items for patients who are or are not MV without testing for equivalency • Studies of the CPOT English version show it discriminates between pain and no pain with a score >3 yielded a sensitivity of 66.7% and specificity of 83.3% during turning for a small population of critically ill mainly head trauma patients; however, the French version has different statistics that English version studies sometimes use • Varying levels of pain have been tested, but unable to be distinguished with the CPOT • Scores are often restricted to the lower end of the scale	• Demonstrates beginning level of clinical usefulness in critically ill patients; further work is suggested in palliative care subjects across settings • Psychometric testing of the Compliance with MV subscale and the Vocalization scale is suggested • Numerous training scenarios reported • Unconventional scoring may lead to misinterpretation • Some items may need additional work to ease interpretation • Time between training and implementation should be short • Comparisons needed between the French and English versions, including additional work on sensitivity and specificity

	compliance feedback sent to users, posted, discussed at staff meetings, and incorporated into individual performance reviews	• Infrequent use may affect clinical usefulness perceptions • Implementation significantly increased pain assessments • Analgesic and sedative use, ICU duration of stay and duration of MV findings were inconsistent		• Pain assessment findings should be paired with analgesic orders
FLACC[46,53,54]	15 s to 2 min	Raters trained to a target 85% agreement	—	Measures presence of pain, not severity, and uses the familiar 0–10 scale	• Thorough training description and formal clinical usefulness analysis in a variety of settings and populations, including palliative care are suggested • Short administration time • Purported to be widely used in adult critically ill patients, suggesting clinical usefulness, despite lack of a formal clinical usefulness assessment and minimal IR assessment by nurse raters

(continued on next page)

Table 3
(continued)

Tool/Author	Administration Time	Training[a]	Clinical Usefulness[b]	Score Interpretation[c]	Comments
MOPAT[56–61] (McGuire, personal communication, 2016)	1 min observation time plus scoring (McGuire, personal communication, 2016)	• Mandatory training using videotapes with pre-determined consensus ratings, with or without bedside demonstrations, with or without unit based nurse champions • Requested and responded to formal and informal feedback from nurse users • For longitudinal use, compliance auditing with frequent feedback (individual user level and aggregate unit level data) with documentation requirement reminders, screen shots, and flyers	• An overwhelming majority of nurses (with or without licensed practical nurses) across settings reported that the MOPAT took a reasonable time to complete, was easy to use, was helpful in assessing pain, was helpful in determining the presence of pain or if an intervention was needed, and assisted in communicating about pain • A majority to overwhelming majority reported it was feasible to (or they would) use the MOPAT in their clinical setting and that informal care givers could use it with training	• Assesses presence of pain, not severity (in recent unpublished findings, levels indicative of mild, moderate, and severe pain have been established) • Sensory dimension was not often used, and has been deleted from the current version • Physiologic dimension differ in acute care and hospice versions • Physiologic dimension is not scored in the current AC version and is under revision • Integrated into EHR in an inpatient hospice and AMC • Uses a 0–12 scale, different from frequently used self-report scales • There are scoring differences for the acute care and hospice versions	• Thorough training description for hospice and acute care (training in an non-study outpatient hospice setting also described) • Formal clinical usefulness analysis in acute care and hospice settings demonstrates good to excellent clinical usefulness when used with palliative care in-patients, including the critically ill, traumatic brain injury, and patients at the end of life • All studies used registered nurse with or without licensed practical nurse raters, demonstrating the MOPAT is appropriate for nurses' use • Uses a 0–12 scale, different from frequently used self-report scales • Testing recommended in informal caregivers

NCS[62-64]	10–60 s during spontaneous eye opening, to ensure a sufficient level of arousal	—	• Scores range from 0 to 12 • A score of 4 did not discriminate well between pain and no pain	• Determine ideal observation time • Specify training • Cut scores indicative of no pain and pain states need validation • Assess clinical usefulness
Revised NCS[65,66]	10–60 s of observation excluding scoring, with more behaviors seen after longer observation periods	2 h training with a video session	• Scores range 0–9 • A score of 3 or 4 respectively, may discriminate between pain and no pain in patients in a vegetative or minimally conscious state; further testing is suggested	• The 0–9 scale is different from frequently used self-report scales • Needs testing to determine scores indicative of none, mild, moderate, and severe pain • Cut scores indicative of no pain and pain states need validation • Observation periods need standardization • Clinical usefulness assessment is needed • Comparisons between the NCS and revised NCS should be performed

(continued on next page)

Table 3
(continued)

Tool/Author	Administration Time	Training[a]	Clinical Usefulness[b]	Score Interpretation[c]	Comments
NVPS[49,54,68–70]	15 s observation time (Marmo)	• Comprehensive educational programs (eg, 15–20 min) that may include the following rationale for tool implementation, demonstration, practice sessions with 85%–90% interrater agreement, and use of documentation tool • Bedside aids often used (laminated cards and/or posters containing the tool, pain policy assessment reminders, graphics of behaviors) • Additional clinical implementation suggestions: planning, staff involvement/motivation, regular monitoring and feedback by a designated change agent and problem solver	• In 100 ratings, only 1 individual NVPS item was deemed not applicable once • An overwhelming majority of nurses found it easy to use and were satisfied/very satisfied with training • Compared with preimplementation, postimplementation nurses felt it improved their confidence in assessing unconscious patients' pain, but there was no change in their confidence about managing pain • After NVPS implementation, nurses were significantly less likely to agree that an appropriate pain score would ease assessment, make them more confident in requesting more or less analgesia, or improve their pain management practices	• Assesses presence of pain, not pain severity, but no testing has been done to determine the score that distinguishes between no pain and pain • Scores range from 0 to 10 • Some researchers, other than the developers, have identified anchors for the top and bottom of the scale (eg, no pain and maximal pain) without statistical validation	• Although no information was provided about the time required for administration, nurses reported it easy to use and were satisfied with the training • Studies provide numerous training program descriptions that focus on clinical implementation and bedside aids that are likely applicable to other behaviorally based pain assessment tools

NVPS-R[27,48,69,70]	—	• Training session (<1 h) with or without with demonstration, tool practice session or 90% interrater agreement • Clinical implementation suggestions: planning, staff involvement and motivation, training, resources (laminated cards with tool and pain assessment policy reminders), regular monitoring and feedback by a designated change agent/problem solver	• Quick and easy to use, simple to understand, easy to complete • Median score 7–8 (0 = worst, 10 = best) for accuracy, usefulness, and ease of learning • Although there was not a significant difference, nurses had a greater preference for the NVPS (43%) compared with BPS (33%) and CPOT (24%), but preference could be related to previous familiarity	See NVPS	• See NVPS • Clinical usefulness comparisons between the NVPS and NVPS-R are needed

Administration time is the approximate amount of time required for tool completion.

Training is the specifics about training used in studies (eg, amount of time, type of training, resources used).

Abbreviations: BPS, Behavioral Pain Scale; BPS-NI, Behavioral Pain Scale for nonintubated patients with delirium; CNPI, Checklist of Nonverbal Pain Indicators; CPOT, Critical Care Pain Observation Tool; EHR, electronic health record; ICU, intensive care unit; FLACC, Faces, Legs, Activity, Cry, Consolability; MOPAT, Multidimensional Observational Pain Assessment Tool; MV, mechanical ventilation; NCS, Nociceptive Coma Scale; NRS, numerical rating scale; NVPS, Nonverbal Pain Scale; NVPS-R, Revised Nonverbal Pain Scale.

[a] Study-related training is not described and if a training time reported by the authors included study procedures, a < sign was placed in front of the time indicating that actual clinical training time will be less.

[b] Clinical usefulness includes specific information about the usefulness, advantages and disadvantages of the tool or associated documentation process.

[c] Sensitivity refers to the ability to correctly detect people who are experiencing pain; specificity refers to the ability to identify those who are not experiencing pain.

Advanced Dementia,[33] including the general palliative care population. The CNPI has been incorporated into electronic medical record systems and used with palliative care patients in an acute care hospital[34] and a hospice setting,[35] suggesting that clinicians find it useful in these environments.

Critical Care Pain Observation Tool

The Critical Care Pain Observation Tool (CPOT) was originally developed in French for assessing pain in hospitalized critically ill ventilated patients. It consisted of 4 behavioral categories: (1) facial expression, (2) body movements, (3) muscle tension, and (4) compliance with mechanical ventilators (for ventilated patients) or vocalization (for extubated patients), each of which is scored on a 0 to 2 scale of various verbal descriptors, with a possible total score ranging from 0 to 8.[36] The effect of the 2 different items (mechanical ventilation compliance and vocalization) have not been explored.

A follow-up study[37] evaluated the English version of the CPOT in conscious (with varying levels of ability to self-report) and unconscious critically ill ventilated patients, focusing on reliability and validity, and also examined physiologic indicators thought to be associated with pain (mean arterial pressure, heart rate, respiratory rate, and transcutaneous oxygen saturation). Results demonstrated that the CPOT was reliable and valid and that physiologic indicators were not correlated with self-report of pain, leading to a suggestion that they be used as a cue to perform a behavioral pain assessment. This suggestion was subsequently echoed by Chen and Chen[38] when trying to validate physiologic indicators (vital signs) for pain assessment and is consistent with the American Society for Pain Management Nursing Practice Guidelines.[2]

Sensitivity and specificity of the CPOT has been assessed in the English[37] and French[39] versions, with varying results, potentially attributable to differences in language or populations, but additional testing is needed. A large proportion of nurses who used the CPOT reported that the instructions were clear and that they found it simple to use, easy to understand, and helpful for their practice.[40] Use of the CPOT had positive effects on nurses' pain assessment and documentation, and may affect treatment processes, mechanical ventilation time, and intensive care unit duration of stay,[41] but its effects on patients' pain outcomes remain to be evaluated. The CPOT's reliability and validity have been confirmed in several small studies conducted by other investigators,[42,43] although one[42] noted lower interrater reliability than initial studies and suggested the use of standardized instructions and training. Others have extended the use of the CPOT to neurologic intensive care unit patients who had brain surgery[44] and critically ill patients with delirium,[45] but unfortunately both French and English versions were used and treated as one in the analysis. Specific details about the translation have not been provided. Because neurosurgical and delirium populations are frequently encountered in critical care and palliative care patient populations, these studies should be replicated removing the confounder of language. Numerous investigators have conducted studies comparing the CPOT to other behavioral pain assessment tools in intensive care units of various types.[18,27,46–48] In most studies, the CPOT performed as well as or better than other tools, although it did not perform well in a burn population, which could self-report.[49] It is noteworthy that none of the initial or subsequent CPOT psychometric studies used samples that were exclusively nonverbal, and furthermore, frequently used the traditional gold standard comparison with self-report measures when assessing concurrent validity. Because noncommunicative patients may show more pain behaviors than those who are communicative, the effects of these methodologic differences are unknown.[30,50] The CPOT has the largest body of research supporting its development and similar to the BPS, has been recommended for use in adult critical care settings in postoperative, medical or trauma (except for brain injury) patients who cannot self-report but who have intact motor function and observable behaviors.[25] Its versatility as a pain assessment tool across palliative care settings and patients has not yet been examined.

Face, Legs, Activity, Cry, and Consolability Pain Tool

The Faces, Legs, Activity, Cry, Consolability (FLACC) pain tool originated in the pediatric population as a simple measure of pain severity.[51] The FLACC scores each of 5 behaviors (face, legs, activity, cry, consolability) on a scale from 0 (normal or no findings) to 2 (frequent and intense behaviors) for an overall score of 0 to 10.[52] Although the FLACC was developed and tested in children, a paucity of evidence exists for its use in adults. Voepel-Lewis and colleagues[53] conducted a subsequent study in a small sample of critically ill adults (n = 29) and children (n = 8) who could not self-report. Using the CNPI (for adults) or the Comfort Scale (for children) as the gold standard, they found acceptable and significant correlations with the FLACC. However, no gold standard has been identified for observational pain scales, the CNPI does not have robust evidence for reliability and validity, and the Comfort scale assesses sedation and pain as a combined construct. Interrater reliability was reported separately for both the adult and pediatric population and the FLACC showed higher levels of agreement for each of the items and the overall tool compared with the pediatric population. Factor analysis and discriminant validity were reported for the combined adult and pediatric population, making it impossible to discern how the FLACC performed in the adult population. Based on the combined sample data, the authors suggested that the FLACC might be useful across populations and settings. Two studies, one comparing the FLACC with the CPOT and Nonverbal Pain Scale (NVPS; see below),[54] and the other comparing the FLACC with the CPOT[46] inexplicably omitted data on the FLACC and focused almost exclusively on the CPOT, thus adding little to knowledge about the FLACC. Although Buttes and colleagues[46] noted that the 2 study data collectors thought the CPOT was more appropriate for adults than the FLACC, they did not present an explanation to support this statement. With minimal empirical data on the reliability, validity, and clinical usefulness of the FLACC pain tool in adult populations, particularly those in palliative care, it is unclear whether the FLACC is suitable for assessing pain in adults in palliative care across settings and further study is warranted.

Multidimensional Observational Pain Assessment Tool

The Multidimensional Observational Pain Assessment Tool (MOPAT) was adapted from the PACU [postanesthesia care unit] Behavioral Pain Rating Scale.[55] The MOPAT was modified to serve as a measure of 2 dimensions of pain (behavioral and physiologic) that could be used in noncommunicative individuals across palliative care settings. In the original formulation, the developers included a third dimension, sensory, focusing on the temporal pattern of pain.[56] The behavioral dimension is composed of 4 behaviors scored on a scale of 0 (no behavior displayed) to 3 (most severe behavior): (1) restlessness, (2) tense muscles, (3) frowning/grimacing, and (4) patient sounds, which are summed for a behavioral dimension score ranging from 0 to 12. The MOPAT uses a substitution formula in patients who cannot make any sounds.

The physiologic dimension is composed of 4 physiologic indicators: (1) blood pressure, (2) heart rate, (3) respirations, and (4) diaphoresis, each scored dichotomously, with 0 indicating normal or no change from the patient's baseline, and 1 indicating abnormal or a change from baseline, summed for a physiologic dimension score ranging from 0 to 4. These 2 dimension scores are then summed for a total MOPAT score ranging from 0 to 16. The sensory dimension is designed to assess pattern of pain by using behavioral and physiologic ratings over time, in conjunction with knowledge of pain etiology, to choose among 3 groups of adjectives adapted from the McGill Pain Questionnaire Long Form (brief/momentary/transient; rhythmic/periodic/intermittent; continuous/steady/constant). Several small-scale developmental studies that were conducted in inpatient hospice settings demonstrated initial evidence of reliability, validity, and clinical usefulness of the behavioral and physiologic dimensions, but little use of the sensory dimension.[56] These results led to full-scale psychometric evaluation of a revised MOPAT consisting of behavioral and physiologic dimensions in both the acute care hospital and inpatient hospice settings. In the latter setting, the blood pressure item was eliminated from the physiologic scale because blood pressure monitoring causes pain and is generally not done in hospice settings. This altered format changed the score on the physiologic dimension to a range of 0 to 3 and the MOPAT total score to a range of 0 to 15 in the hospice population.[57] All patients in the study were completely noncommunicative, but the different versions of the tool were appropriately tested separately. The acute care hospital sample was primarily from critical care units, although some patients were on regular inpatient units. Data from both settings yielded evidence of reliability, validity, and clinical usefulness when the MOPAT was used cross-sectionally (before or after a pain intervention)[58] and longitudinally in the acute care hospital (Wiegand DL, Wilson T, Pannullo D, et al. Measuring acute pain in the critically ill. Unpublished data), and longitudinally in the inpatient hospice setting.[57,59]

Based on the findings, the physiologic dimension has undergone some changes. The diaphoresis item has been dropped from the hospice version and is no longer scored in the acute care setting (McGuire, personal communication, 2016). Further exploratory work on this dimension in the acute care setting is underway.[60] The MOPAT has been incorporated into several electronic health record systems and is currently used as the standard of care pain assessment tool for noncommunicative palliative care patients in a hospice and an acute care hospital.[57,59,61] Because the MOPAT was not tested in patients with dementia, it is not recommended for use in that group. Ongoing research is examining the helpfulness of the MOPAT in reducing pain and improving pharmacologic management as part of a comprehensive algorithm/order set for palliative care patients in the acute care setting.

Nociceptive Coma Scale

The Nociceptive Coma Scale (NCS) was developed initially in Belgium as a means to assess nociception (used as a proxy for pain) in patients who were in a vegetative state or minimally conscious state and unable to self-report their pain.[62] The NCS includes 4 items: (1) motor response, (2) verbal response, (3) visual response, and (4) facial expression, each scored from 0 to 3, with 0 representing none and 3 representing what seem to be increased response levels, for example, "localization to noxious stimulation" for motor response, or "fixation" for visual response. The NCS is a new albeit behaviorally based approach to pain assessment in a specific medical situation (ie, coma) that is arguably somewhat different from the typical noncommunicative population. Initial testing compared the NCS with several well-known behavioral pain assessment tools (eg, CNPI, FLACC, Pain Assessment in Advanced Dementia), demonstrating validity, reliability, and sensitivity. Scores were higher in patients in a minimally conscious state, suggesting the tool's adaptability for assessing nociception in disorders of consciousness. Although the authors used an experimental pain model, they recommended the tool for following patients' behaviors and monitoring treatments to avoid overtreatment or undertreatment.

Subsequent research using an experimental pain model demonstrated test–retest reliability[63] and more fully assessed the sensitivity of the NCS by comparing behavioral changes in response to noxious or nonnoxious stimulation.[64] Observing that the verbal response item was not sensitive and, when eliminated, almost doubled the sensitivity of the NCS to different levels of consciousness, the investigators created the revised NCS, which omitted the verbal response item. While acknowledging the lack of psychometric data for the revised NCS, the authors nonetheless concluded (based on the initial validation work) that the revised NCS was valid and sensitive in patients with disorders of consciousness.

Another outcome of this study was the identification of a potential cutoff value of 4 for minimally conscious state and 3 for patients in a vegetative state who distinguished noxious from nonnoxious stimulation. In more recent research that induced experimental pain, Chatelle and colleagues[65] used PET studies to demonstrate a significant positive correlation between revised NCS scores and glucose metabolism in the anterior cingulate cortex, which is involved in pain processing. They concluded that the revised NCS total scores are related to cortical processing and are, therefore, an appropriate mechanism for assessing, monitoring, and treating "possible" pain in patients with disorders of consciousness. It is unknown if there would be differences in psychometric findings for clinical pain. One subsequent clinical study demonstrated a significant decrease in revised NCS scores after analgesic administration and suggested further exploration of using 4 as an revised NCS cutoff value to determine analgesic treatment.[66] This intriguing tool has potential for use in comatose palliative care patients across settings, but clearly needs additional research on psychometric properties and clinical usefulness using clinical populations before any conclusions can be drawn.

Nonverbal Pain Scale

The NVPS was initially developed to assess pain in adult patients on a burn trauma unit.[67] It was "patterned after the FLACC, but modified to reflect assessment components more appropriate to an adult population."[67]. Specifically, the NVPS eliminated the legs, cry, and consolability components of the FLACC, retained and revised the face and activity components, and added 3 items identified in previous research as being related to pain or its control: (1) guarding, (2) physiologic 1 (vital signs), and (3) physiologic 2 (skin, pupils, perspiration, flushing, diaphoresis, pallor). The physiologic 1 component included specific numeric values for vital signs (eg, heart rate of more than 20 or 25 bpm during the previous 4 hours) that were considered evidence of pain, although the rationale was not elucidated.[67] The FLACC's 3-point scoring system (0–2 range for each component) was retained for the NVPS. The scores for each of the 5 NVPS components are summed for a total score of 0 to 10. The study compared the NVPS to the FLACC in entirely noncommunicative burn, abdominal surgery, and trauma patients who might potentially have pain. The study provided evidence of discriminant validity for the NVPS, and provided some evidence of the FLACC's limitations for use in adults related to the cry and consolability items. The authors observed that the physiologic 1 indicator significantly influenced the total score, whereas the physiologic 2 indicator was only moderately correlated, perhaps because its components were somewhat subjective (eg, dilated pupils). Although the authors suggested the tool was reliable, no results were provided. Clinical usefulness was also not assessed formally in the study.

Topolovec-Vranik and colleagues[68] examined the clinical usefulness of the original NVPS by exploring patient satisfaction and documentation of pain assessment and management in a trauma/neurosurgery intensive care unit before, during, and after implementation of the NVPS. Although patient satisfaction was not significantly different in the preimplementation and postimplementation groups, patient reports of worst pain significantly decreased after implementation, and there was a clinically significant trend in decrease of severe pain and time to receive pain medications. The authors noted that these findings could be related to differences in characteristics of the 2 groups. Staff nurses found the NVPS easy to use, were more confident in assessing pain in nonverbal sedated patients, were satisfied with the training they received, and were more satisfied in the approach to managing patients' pain. Nurses' documentation of pain assessment increased significantly in noncommunicative patients; however, no differences in treatment were noted. Although this study was intended to explore what happened when the NPVS was initiated, the direct impact on patient outcomes was difficult to ascertain.

Comparisons of the NPVS with the CPOT revealed poorer interrater reliability in a burn population that included patients who could self-report.[49] The NPVS underwent a revision early in its development, as evidenced in a short publication in which Wegman[69] provided a visual depiction of the NVPS and noted the transformation of the poorly performing physiologic 2 to an item called *respiratory*. Kabes and colleagues[70] conducted a comparison study of the NVPS and the NVPS-R in adult intensive care unit patients who were unable to verbalize pain, mechanically ventilated, and sedated. Their results demonstrated that the NVPS-R was reliable, valid, and in general performed better because of the respiratory item. Subsequent studies have compared the psychometric properties of the NVPS-R with various forms of the CPOT and the BPS in several populations. In general, the NVPS-R did not perform as well as the other tools or sometimes did not meet acceptable levels,[27,48,71] demonstrating that the NVPS-R may need additional work. There is little evidence that the NPVS or the NPVS-R has been used in palliative care populations or settings, and there are ongoing concerns about reliability, validity, and clinical usefulness. More work is warranted to distinguish between the 2 versions, and to clarify their psychometric properties, appropriate use, and impact on clinical outcomes.

KEY FACTORS IN SELECTING PAIN ASSESSMENT TOOLS

Consistent use of a reliable, valid, and clinically useful pain assessment allows for identification of pain, evaluation of treatments, and communication among health care providers and families. It is a first step toward improving outcomes and begins with the selection of an appropriate tool. Selection of a pain assessment tool for use in a specific setting and population is an important undertaking because a good fit between the tool and the setting is critical for uptake and improvement in pain-related outcomes. The numerous factors that should be considered in this decision process in any setting[4,13,72] are shown in **Table 4**, with a few factors discussed in more detail because they are especially germane to successful implementation of any pain assessment tool.

When selecting a tool, review articles such as this one may help to narrow the field. When reviewing a tool, it is important to understand that published reliability and validity data are generated from a specific version of a pain assessment tool (see **Table 2**). If a tool is changed, then the psychometric parameters need to be reassessed. Without reliability and validity data from a population and setting similar to the user's, it is unknown if the tool is assessing pain as intended or whether different raters obtain the same response. These issues can cause measurement error and affect the pain ratings in unknown ways.

Although there is no consensus on the components of clinical usefulness, it is also an important parameter to consider. Clinical usefulness refers to the usefulness, advantages, and disadvantages of a new technique, technology, or intervention and

Table 4	
Factors to consider when selecting a pain assessment tool for noncommunicative patients	
Factor to Consider	**Why Is It Important?**
Validity	A tool must be valid to measure what it is supposed to measure, be well-founded, and correspond accurately with the real world.
Reliability	A tool must be reliable to produce similar results under consistent conditions, or consistent measures of a particular element over a period of time and between different participants.
Clinical usefulness	The tool needs to be user friendly, acceptable to users, and helpful in managing pain.
Patients and settings	Using a tool in a patient population and setting for which it is intended will enhance appropriate use and produce more valid and reliable assessment data.
Compatibility with, and relevance for, current clinical practice	If a tool is incompatible with practice patterns or preferences, or is viewed as not relevant, it will not be used.
Stakeholders and gate keepers	Individuals who are key to the adoption of a new assessment tool must be supportive so that they can facilitate rather than discourage use of the tool.
Facilitators and barriers	Identification of these factors will enable development of a realistic implementation plan; examples include nurses' beliefs and attitudes, interest in adopting new innovations, commitment to evidence-based practice, etc.
Education and training	Resources for education and training for adoption of a new tool must be available; compatibility with existing in-service educational systems is essential.
Documentation system (eg, electronic health record)	Incorporation into the setting's documentation system is absolutely essential to ensure consistent use.

typically includes such dimensions as appropriateness, accessibility, practicality, feasibility, and acceptability.[17] Similar to reliability and validity, clinical usefulness findings are specific to the version of the tool that was tested (see **Table 3**). A tool that is valid and reliable but has not been examined for clinical usefulness may not perform as desired, nor be attractive to clinicians.

Of particular relevance in the selection of a tool is a review of not only of the original articles, but of comparison studies since they may offer useful information on how tools performed in a specific setting when compared with one another.[27,72] In addition, if clinicians are looking for a tool that can be used across several clinical settings, for example, in an acute care setting followed by inpatient rehabilitation or hospice, they need to determine in what settings a tool was used and how it performed. If a tool looks promising but has not been evaluated in that setting, clinicians may want to consider a quality improvement project or a research study to examine its clinical usefulness in their own setting.

When implementing a new pain assessment tool, it is important to ensure that adequate training and resources are available and to carefully plan a process that includes staff and gets them motivated.[70] Helpful strategies for this process include engaging appropriate committees, enlisting unit-based nurse champions, developing streamlined educational programs that are incorporated into institutional training systems, and mandating the training with clear deadlines for completion.[61] For behavior-based tools, demonstration, practice sessions and an assessment of competency are imperative upon initiation, when training new staff, and as intermittent refreshers to ensure appropriate and consistent use over time by numerous professional caregivers. Bedside tools such as posters, pocket cards, and tip sheets reinforce training and facilitate implementation.[61,68] Periodic retraining may be needed for nurses who use the tool infrequently.

Box 1
Case 1: Neurointensive Care Unit and transfer to Intermediate Care

Part 1: Admission to the Neurointensive Care Unit

Medical Condition: Mr X was hit by a car while jogging and experienced a traumatic injury for which he had a right above-the-knee amputation. He is intubated and noncommunicative when he arrives on the unit. Mr X has a Richmond Agitation Scale Score of −3 (movement or eye opening to voice but no eye contact) and a Glasgow Coma Scale score of 3T (eye opening to pain = 2, verbal response intubated = t; best motor response non/untestable = 1).

Current Pain Situation: Nursing staff has been routinely administering PRN analgesia before turning him, because during earlier turning episodes Mr X was constantly frowning and very tense.

Pain Assessment: The nurse assesses pain using an appropriate reliable and valid tool that indicates the presence of pain.

Vital signs: Blood pressure 155/87, heart rate 115, respiratory rate 20, and presence of diaphoresis.

Pain Intervention: The nurse administers oxycodone via the nasogastric tube.

Pain Reassessment: The nurse returns to assess pain and turn the patient in 60 minutes, the approximate time of peak effect for liquid oxycodone administered via nasogastric tube. The pain score indicates that no pain is present.

Vital signs: blood pressure 104/84, heart rate 94, respiratory rate 16, and no diaphoresis.

Take-Home Message: Pain assessment of noncommunicative patients for the presence or severity of pain with a reliable and valid tool can provide consistency over time. Vital signs may provide a cue that pain is present and/or has been relieved.

Part 2: Transfer to the Neuro Intermediate Care/Step-down Unit

Medical Condition: Mr X has been diagnosed with traumatic brain injury. He is extubated but noncommunicative when transferred. He now has an infection of the amputation incision. His Richmond Agitation Scale Score is +2 agitation (frequent nonpurposeful movement) and his Glasgow Coma Scale is 8 (eye opening score 4-spontaneous, Verbal response score 1 [not testable], and best motor response score 3 [flexes]).

Current Pain Situation: In performing the first dressing change, the nurse notes that Mr X is restless and groaning, so she surmises that he may have procedural pain and stops.

Pain Assessment: The nurse assesses him for pain in preparation for administering pain medication. The pain score indicates the presence of pain.

Vital signs: Blood pressure 149/70, heart rate 100, respiratory rate 20, and no diaphoresis.

Pain Intervention: The nurse administers intravenous hydromorphone before continuing with the dressing change.

Pain Reassessment: The nurse returns to reassess pain in 30 minutes, the approximate time of peak effect for intravenous hydromorphone. Reassessment with the pain tool indicates that no pain is present when the patient is at rest, so the nurse completes the dressing change and modifies the pain management plan to include medication before dressing changes.

Vital signs: Blood pressure 123/69, heart rate 69, respiratory rate 11, and no diaphoresis.

Take Home Message: Pain assessment and reassessment using the same reliable and valid pain assessment tool across clinical settings can help enhance communication among different health care personnel and enable revision of the pain management plan as needed.

Incorporating the tool into the institution's documentation system (eg, electronic health record), and monitoring use and outcomes via a quality improvement process or research study is essential for successful implementation of the tool.[34,61] Because clinical implementation involves the use of a tool in real patients, it is

---

Box 2
Case 2: Medical Intensive Care Unit and transfer to Inpatient Hospice

Part 1: Medical Intensive Care Unit

Medical Condition: Mrs Y has been hospitalized for a month with acute respiratory distress syndrome, chronic obstructive pulmonary disease, and history of rheumatoid arthritis, has a tracheostomy tube, and is on a ventilator. Weaning off the ventilator has been unsuccessful. She continues to deteriorate and has developed acute kidney failure requiring dialysis. A family meeting is held and the patient's advance directive (AD) was reviewed in relation to her current status. The AD and Medical Orders for Life-Sustaining Treatment state that the patient wanted a trial on the ventilator support and dialysis, but would not want to be sustained by these treatments indefinitely.

Current Pain Situation: The nursing staff has been administering analgesics routinely before suctioning because Mrs Y was exhibiting restlessness and body arching when suctioned. The nurse plans to medicate the patient for anticipated procedural pain before suctioning.

Pain Assessment: The nurse assesses Mrs Y with a reliable and valid pain tool before administering pain medication, observing mild restlessness and frowning.

Vital signs: Blood pressure 130/66, heart rate 104, respiratory rate 12, no diaphoresis.

Pain Intervention: Based on the patient's previous response to suctioning and consultation with the respiratory therapist, the nurse administers intravenous hydromorphone to prepare for suctioning.

Reassessment: The nurse returns in 30 minutes, which is the approximate time of peak effect for intravenous hydromorphone. Assessment with the pain tool demonstrates that no pain is present, and the respiratory therapist suctions the patient. Directly after the suctioning, the nurse reassesses the patient and observes no signs of pain.

Vital signs: Blood pressure 120/70, heart rate 100, respiratory rate 11, no diaphoresis.

Take Home Message: Preemptive pain assessment and intervention for procedures that are known to cause pain improves pain management and patient comfort.

Part 2: Transfer to Inpatient Hospice

Medical Condition: Mrs Y has been hospitalized for 5 weeks. Based on the AD, she was taken off the ventilator and dialysis was stopped. She is in a semicomatose state and has been transferred to inpatient hospice.

Pain Assessment: The nursing staff has been routinely assessing for pain every 2 hours using a reliable and valid tool. On one of the assessments, Mrs Y is very restless and tense.

Vital signs: Blood pressure 140/80, heart rate 90, respiratory rate 22, diaphoresis present.

Pain Intervention: The nurse administers oxycodone liquid via the gastrostomy tube.

Pain Reassessment: The nurse returns in 60 minutes, which is the approximate time of peak effect for liquid oxycodone administered via gastrointestinal tube. The pain tool shows moderate restlessness and frowning, so the nurse gives another dose, per existing orders. She returns in 60 minutes and finds the patient calm and relaxed.

Vital signs: Blood pressure 136/78, heart rate 86, respiratory rate 18, no diaphoresis.

Take Home Message: Some reliable and valid behavioral pain assessment tools are able to assess both presence and severity of pain. Pain-related behaviors may change over time. Vital signs may or may not fluctuate with different levels of pain severity. Routine use of a pain assessment tool can help to identify episodes of breakthrough pain, thereby facilitating optimal pain management.

important to establish specific targets and methods to achieve them. Tracking nurses' use and documentation of the tool via audits and providing data-based feedback at the unit and user level are some ways to assess uptake and adherence.[6,34,35,41,61,68]

Finally, determining nurses' perceptions of benefits and potential effects on their practice patterns, as well as enlisting their feedback, facilitates nurses' involvement in the practice change, an important change strategy, and also helps to identify problematic areas so that timely corrections can be initiated.[61] Measuring relevant outcomes such as frequency of assessment may be more helpful than trying to gauge increases or decreases in administration of pain medications.[41] It is also important to link assessment results with pain management interventions through the development of algorithms that incorporate the pain assessment tool and specify scores or cutpoints that trigger pain interventions[26,73] and to consider outcomes such as patient or family caregiver satisfaction.[26,68]

CASE STUDIES

Three case studies are presented to illustrate the variety of noncommunicative palliative care patients and settings for whom pain assessment is needed. Details of each case's medical condition, pain situation, pain assessment, treatment, and reassessment are described. The description concludes with a brief take-home message that emphasizes key points related to proper assessment and management of pain in each case. The descriptions are deliberately generic with respect to the pain assessment tools used; thus, readers are encouraged to select and use a pain assessment tool of their choice when reading through the cases. This exercise may be helpful in exploring the potential use of one of the pain assessment tools described in this paper or in confirming one that is already used in the reader's setting (**Boxes 1–3**).

Box 3
Case 3: Inpatient hospice

Medical Condition: Ms Z has lung cancer, is nonresponsive, and is bed bound.

Current Pain Situation: Three hours ago, the nurse attempted to turn Ms Z, but when she was moved, she frowned and groaned softly and her body became very stiff. Ms Z's usual vital signs were heart rate 90, respiratory rate 10, and no diaphoresis, but when she was moved her heart rate was 122, respiratory rate 24, and she became diaphoretic. Because these behaviors and changes in vital signs may indicate pain, the nurse premedicated her before moving her again, but observes stiffness.

Pain Assessment: The nurse uses a valid and reliable tool that is integrated into the electronic health record to enable a standardized pain assessment. Ms Z has a pain score that indicates pain is present.

Pain Intervention: The nurse administers oxycodone via a nasogastric tube, turns the patient, and provides a backrub.

Pain Reassessment: The nurse reassess pain after this multimodal intervention using the same tool, and determines that no pain is present.

Take Home Message: Some pain assessment tools are effective for assessing both pharmacologic and nonpharmacologic interventions. Incorporation into the electronic health record standardizes pain assessment and enables timely interventions.

SUMMARY

Use of a valid, reliable, and clinically useful behavioral based pain assessment tool for adult noncommunicative palliative care patients is only one aspect of pain assessment, and should be combined with a comprehensive pain assessment.[4] However, there are limitations to the use of behavioral based tools that need to be considered. Patients who can provide some level of self-report may display fewer behaviors, raising questions about appropriateness of behavioral based tools for this group. In some patients, a physical examination may need to be coupled with a pain assessment, for example, in patients with visceral pain, to obtain useful data. In other patients, it may be difficult to distinguish pain from anxiety, so again, using other techniques and information about the patient may be helpful.

There are many patient groups for whom there are no good tools, for example, patients receiving paralytic agents or who are paralyzed, those with chronic/persistent pain, or those with traumatic brain injury or other neurologic impairments. Most tools have not been tested in patients who go in and out of noncommunicative states, and thus have variable abilities to self-report. When physiologic variables are included in a tool, users need to be aware of previous research suggesting that they are questionable.[54] Many of the tools tested in intubated critically ill patients have not been tested in nonintubated patients.[27] In addition, some conditions may mute behavioral responses, for example, anesthesia,[42] and sedatives and other medications.[40]

Few behavioral tools can determine level of pain (mild, moderate, severe) because they have not been tested for this function. When using any of these tools, it is important to be able to score the patient on all the tool's items.[4] Some patients may need to be moved or experience a painful procedure to mount a response that can be scored with a behavioral tool.[34] Tools with lower reliability and validity may not be as sensitive when patients are at rest.[71] Moreover, not all studies report data on reliability and validity scores at rest and movement, and sometimes scores at rest are lower. Once a tool is complete, it is important to realize that the score cannot be interpreted in the same way as self-report scores, which generally use a continuous scale.[71] Finally, researchers do not always report which version of a tool they are testing, requiring the clinician to try and make this determination.

Although this review has provided helpful information about behavior-based pain assessment tools in adult palliative care noncommunicative patients, it has also revealed numerous areas for further work. Studies are needed on how pain assessment tools can be used for treatment decision making, and which scores may actually indicate pain versus other phenomena. More research is needed in a variety of patient populations and settings. The effects of small but significant differences in psychometric properties of tools are unknown, as is how these might affect patient outcomes.[27] When a patient's credibility in self-reporting is unclear, it may be helpful to add a behavior-based tool; however, there is little research in this area so the implications for practice are unknown. Even with these limitations, the tools reviewed herein do offer potential ways to assess pain in the vulnerable population of adult noncommunicative palliative care patients, enabling nurses in various settings to make headway in improving reducing pain and improving quality of life.

ACKNOWLEDGMENTS

The authors thank Roy Brown, MLIS, AHIP, Tompkins-McCaw Library for the Health Sciences, Virginia Commonwealth University, for his expertise and assistance in the literature search and retrieval process. They also acknowledge Sue Gutkin, MS, RN, Stephanie Leimenstoll, BSN, RN, Richard Shrout, MSN, RN, and Lisa Sullivan,

MSN, RN, for assistance in analyzing some of the pain assessment tools. The contributions of Deb Bortle, MS, RN, and Joan Harrold, MD, MPH, of Hospice & Community Care, Lancaster, PA, to the development of case study three are much appreciated. This work was supported in part by research grants from the National Institute of Nursing Research, National Institutes of Health, Bethesda, MD (5R01NR009684, D.B. McGuire, Principal Investigator; 5R01NR013664, D.B. McGuire and C. B. Shanholtz, Multiple Principal Investigators).

REFERENCES

1. International Association for the Study of Pain (IASP). IASP Taxonomy. 1994. Available at: www.iasp-pain.org/Taxonomy/. Accessed April 1, 2016.
2. Reynolds J, Drew D, Dunwoody C. American society for pain management nursing position statement: pain management at the end of life. Pain Manag Nurs 2013;14(3):172–5.
3. World Health Organization. Palliative care fact sheet N°402. 2015. Available at: www.who.int/mediacentre/factsheets/fs402/en/#. Accessed April 1, 2016.
4. Herr K, Coyne PJ, McCaffrey M, et al. Pain assessment in the patient unable to self-report: position statement with clinical practice recommendations. Pain Manag Nurs 2011;12(4):230–50.
5. The National Consensus Project for Quality Palliative Care. Clinical practice guidelines for quality palliative care, 3rd edition. 2013. Available at: www. nationalconsensusproject.org/guidelines_download2.aspx. Accessed April 4, 2016.
6. Wysong PR. Nurses' beliefs and self-reported practices to pain assessment in nonverbal patients. Pain Manag Nurs 2014;15(1):176–85.
7. Pain info must be conveyed to patients. J Hosp Palliat Nurs 2002;4(1):14–5.
8. Joint Commission Electronic Accreditation Manual: Hospitals. 2015. Available at: www.jointcommission.org/standards_information/edition.aspx. Accessed January 4, 2016.
9. City of Hope Pain and Palliative Care Resource Center. Resources for Pain, Palliative Care, Quality of Life and Cancer Survivorship. 2016. Available at: http://prc.coh.org/. Accessed April 1, 2016.
10. HPNA Position Statement. Available at: http://hpna.advancingexpertcare.org/wp-content/uploads/2015/08/Pain-Management.pdf. Accessed April 1, 2016.
11. McGuire DB, Kim H-J, Lang X. Measuring pain. In: Frank-Stromborg M, Olsen SJ, editors. Instruments for clinical health-care research. 3rd edition. Sudbury (MA): Jones & Bartlett; 2004. p. 603–44.
12. Herr K. Pain in the older adult: an imperative across all health care settings. Pain Manag Nurs 2010;11(2):S1–10.
13. Herr K, Bursch H, Ersek M, et al. Use of pain-behavioral assessment tools in the nursing home. J Gerontol Nurs 2010;36(3):18–29.
14. Cade CH. Clinical tools for the assessment of pain in sedated critically ill adults. Nurs Crit Care 2008;13(6):288–97.
15. Gélinas C, Loiselle C, LeMay S, et al. Theoretical, psychometric, and pragmatic issues in pain measurement. Pain Manag Nurs 2008;9(3):120–30.
16. Payen J-F, Chanques G, Mantz J, et al. Current practices in sedation and analgesia for mechanically ventilated critically ill patients. Anesthesiology 2007; 106(4):687–95.
17. Smart A. A multi-dimensional model of clinical utility. Int J Qual Health Care 2006; 18(5):377–82.

18. Stites M. Observational pain scales in critically ill adults. Crit Care Nurse 2013; 33(3):68–78.

19. Payen J-F, Bru O, Bosson JL, et al. Assessing pain in critically ill sedated patients by using a Behavioral Pain Scale. Crit Care Med 2001;29(12):2258–63.

20. Ahlers S, van Gulik L, van der Veen A, et al. Comparison of different pain scoring systems in critically ill patients in a general ICU. Crit Care 2008;12(1):R15.

21. Aissaoui Y, Zeggwagh AA, Zekraoui A. Validation of a Behavioral Pain Scale in critically ill, sedated, and mechanically ventilated patients. Anesth Analg 2005; 101(5):1470–6.

22. Young J, Sifflett J, Nicoletti S, et al. Use of Behavioral Pain Scale to assess pain in ventilated, unconscious and/or sedated patients. Intensive Crit Care Nurs 2006; 22:32–9.

23. Ahlers SJ, van der Veen AM, van Dijik M, et al. The use of Behavioral Pain Scale to assess pain in conscious sedated patients. Anesth Analg 2010;110(1):127–33.

24. Rahu MA, Grap MJ, Ferguson P, et al. Validity and sensitivity of 6 pain scales in critically ill, intubated adults. Am J Crit Care 2015;24(6):514–24.

25. Barr J, Fraser G, Puntillo K, et al. Clinical Practice Guidelines for the Management of Pain, Agitation, and Delirium in Adults Patients in the Intensive Care Unit. Crit Care Med 2013;41(1):263–306.

26. Chanques G, Jaber S, Barbotte E, et al. Impact of systematic evaluation of pain and agitation in an intensive care unit. Crit Care Med 2006;34(6):1691–9.

27. Chanques G, Pohlman A, Kress J, et al. Psychometric comparison of three behavioural scales for the assessment of pain in critically ill patients unable to self-report. Crit Care 2014;18(R160):12.

28. Chanques G, Payen J-F, Mercier G, et al. Assessing pain in non-intubated critically ill patients unable to self report: an adaptation of the Behavioral Pain Scale. Intensive Care Med 2009;35:2060–7.

29. Feldt K, Ryden MB, Miles S. Treatment of pain in cognitively impaired compared with cognitively intact older patients with hip-fracture. J Am Geriatr Soc 1998;46: 1079–85.

30. Feldt KS. The Checklist of Nonverbal Pain Indicators (CNPI). Pain Manag Nurs 2000;1(1):13–21.

31. City of Hope Pain and Palliative Care Resource Center. Resources for pain, palliative care, quality of life and cancer survivorship Checklist of Nonverbal Pain Indicators review. Available at: http://prc.coh.org/PainNOA/CNPI_D.pdf. Accessed April 1, 2016.

32. Jones KR, Fink R, Hutt E, et al. Measuring pain intensity in nursing home residents. J Pain Symptom Manage 2005;30(6):519–27.

33. Ersek M, Herr K, Neradilek NB, et al. Comparing the psychometric properties of the Checklist of Nonverbal Pain Indicators (CNPI) and the Pain Assessment in Advanced Dementia (PAIN-AD) instruments. Pain Med 2010;11:395–404.

34. Kaiser K. Use of electronic medical records in pain management. In: Pasero C, McCaffery M, editors. Pain management: assessment and pharmacologic management. Baltimore (MD): Mosby; 2011. p. 837–57.

35. Covington-East C, Best J, Hines A. Improving electronic documentation of pain management in nonverbal or cognitively impaired outpatient hospice patients. J Hosp Palliat Nurs 2014;16(3):182–8.

36. Gélinas C, Fillion L, Puntillo KA, et al. Validation of the Critical-Care Pain Observation Tool in adult patients. Am J Crit Care 2006;15(4):420–7.

37. Gélinas C, Johnston C. Pain assessment in critically ill ventilated adults: validation of the Critical Care Pain Observation Tool and physiologic indicators. Clin J Pain 2007;23(6):497–505.

38. Chen H-J, Chen Y-M. Pain assessment: validation of the physiologic indicators in the ventilated adult patient. Pain Manag Nurs 2015;16(2):105–11.

39. Gélinas C, Harel F, Fillion L, et al. Sensitivity and specificity of the Critical-Care Pain Observation Tool for the detection of pain in intubated adults after cardiac surgery. J Pain Symptom Manage 2009;37(1):58–67.

40. Gélinas C. Nurses' evaluation of the feasibility and clinical utility of the Critical-Care Pain Observation Tool. Pain Manag Nurs 2010;11(2):115–25.

41. Rose L, Haslam L, Dale C, et al. Behavioral pain assessment tool for critically ill adults unable to self-report pain. Am J Crit Care 2013;22(3):246–54.

42. Keane KM. Validity and reliability of the Critical Care Pain Observation Tool: a replication study. Pain Manag Nurs 2013;14(40):e216–25.

43. Linde SM, Badger JM, Machan JT, et al. Reevaluation of the Critical-Care Pain Observation Tool in intubated adults after cardiac surgery. Am J Crit Care 2013;22(6):491–7.

44. Echegaray-Benites C, Kapoustina O, Gélinas C. Validation of the use of the Critical-Care Pain Observation Tool (CPOT) with brain surgery patients in the neurosurgical intensive care unit. Intensive Crit Care Nurs 2013;30:257–65.

45. Kanji S, MacPhee H, Singh A, et al. Validation of the Critical Care Pain Observation Tool in critically ill patients with delirium: a prospective cohort study. Crit Care Med 2016;44(5):943–7. Available at:www.ccmjournal.org.

46. Buttes P, Keal G, Cronin SN, et al. Validation of the Critical-Care Pain Observation Tool in adult critically ill patients. Dimens Crit Care Nurs 2014;33(2):78–81.

47. Paulson-Conger M, Leske J, Maidl C, et al. Comparison of two pain assessment tools in nonverbal critical care patients. Pain Manag Nurs 2011;12(4):218–24.

48. Topolovec-Vranik J, Gélinas C, Li Y, et al. Validation and evaluation of two observational assessment tools in a trauma and neurosurgical intensive care unit. Pain Res Manag 2013;18(6):e107–14.

49. Wibbenmeyer L, Sevier A, Liao J, et al. Evaluation of the usefulness of two established pain assessment tools in a burn population. J Burn Care Res 2011;32: 52–60.

50. Puntillo KA, Miaskowski C, Kehrle K, et al. The relationship between behavioral and physiologic indicators of pain, critical care patients' self-reports of pain, and opioid administration. Crit Care Med 1997;25:1159–66.

51. Merkel S, Voepel-Lewis T, Shayevitz JR, et al. The FLACC: a behavioral scale for scoring postoperative pain in young children. Pediatr Nurs 1997;23(3):293–7.

52. Voepel-Lewis T, Malviya S, Merkel S, et al. Behavioral pain assessment and the Face, Legs, Activity, Cry and Consolability instrument. Expert Rev Pharmacoecon Outcomes Res 2003;3(3):317–25.

53. Voepel-Lewis T, Zanotti J, Dammeyer JA, et al. Reliability and validity of the Face, Legs, Activity, Cry, Consolability (FLACC) behavioral scale in assessing pain in critically ill. Am J Crit Care 2010;19(1):55–62.

54. Marmo L, Fowler S. Pain assessment tool in critically ill post-open-heart population. Pain Manag Nurs 2010;11(3):134–40.

55. Mateo O, Krenzischek D. A pilot study to assess the relationship between behavioral manifestations and self-report of pain in post-anesthesia care unit patients. J Post Anesth Nurs 1992;7(1):15–21.

56. McGuire DB, Reifsnyder J, Soeken K, et al. Assessing pain in nonresponsive hospice patients: development and preliminary testing of the Multidimensional Objective Pain Assessment Tool (MOPAT). J Palliat Med 2011;14(3):287–92.
57. Bortle D, Harrold JK. MOPAT A new tool for assessing pain in hospice patients who can't self-report. In: NHPCO 13th Clinical Team Conference and Pediatric Intensive Proceedings. 2012. Available at: www.nhpco.org/sites/default/files/public/CTC12_4B.ppt. Accessed April 7, 2016.
58. McGuire DB, Kaiser KS, Soeken K, et al. Measuring pain in non-communicative palliative care patients in an acute care setting: psychometric evaluation of the Multidimensional Objective Pain Assessment Tool (MOPAT). J Pain Symptom Manage 2011;41:299–300.
59. McGuire DB, Harrold J, Kaiser K, et al. Measuring pain in non-communicative patients in the inpatient hospice setting: psychometric evaluation of the Multidimensional Objective Pain Assessment Tool (MOPAT). J Pain Symptom Manage 2013; 45(2):403–4.
60. Kaiser KS, Haisfield-Wolfe ME, McGuire DB, et al. Assessment of acute pain using physiologic variables in non-communicative patients: nurses' perspectives. J Pain Symptom Manage 2015;49(2):432.
61. Kaiser KS, McGuire DB, Shanholtz C, et al. Implementing an evidence-based tool for assessing pain in non-communicative palliative care patients: Challenges and solutions. J Pain Symptom Manage 2016;51(2):435–6.
62. Schnakers C, Chatelle C, Vanhaudehuyse A, et al. The Nociceptive Coma Scale: a new tool to assess nociception in disorders of consciousness. Pain 2010;148: 215–9.
63. Riganello F, Cortese MD, Arcuri F, et al. A study of the reliability of the Nociception Coma Scale. Clin Rehabil 2013;29(4):388–93.
64. Chatelle C, Majerus S, Whyte J, et al. A sensitive scale to assess nociceptive pain in patients with disorders of consciousness. J Neurol Neurosurg Psychiatry 2012; 83:1233–7.
65. Chatelle C, Thibaut A, Bruno M-A, et al. Nociception Coma Scale-Revised scores correlated with metabolism in the anterior cingulate cortex. Neurorehabil Neural Repair 2014;28(2):149–52.
66. Chatelle C, De Val MD, Cantano A, et al. Is the Nociceptive Coma Scale-Revised a useful clinical tool for managing pain in patients with disorders of consciousness? Clin J Pain 2016;32(4):321–6.
67. Odhner M, Wegman D, Freeland N, et al. Assessing pain control in nonverbal critically ill adults. Dimens Crit Care Nurs 2003;22(6):260–7.
68. Topolovec-Vranik J, Canzian S, Innis J, et al. Patient satisfaction and documentation of pain assessments and management after implementing the Adult Nonverbal Pain Scale. Am J Crit Care 2010;19(4):345–54.
69. Wegman DA. Tool for pain assessment. Crit Care Nurse 2005;25(1):14–5.
70. Kabes AM, Graves JK, Norris J. Further validation of the nonverbal pain scale in intensive care patients. Crit Care Nurse 2009;29(1):59–66.
71. Juarez P, Baker M, Duey D, et al. Comparison of two pain scales for the assessment of pain in the ventilated adult patient. Dimens Crit Care Nurs 2010;29(6): 307–15.
72. Gélinas C, Puntillo KA, Joffe AM, et al. A validated approach to evaluating psychometric properties of pain assessment tools for use in nonverbal critically ill adults. Semin Respir Crit Care Med 2013;34(2):153–68.
73. Olsen B, Rustoen T, Sandvik L, et al. Development of a pain management algorithm for intensive care units. Heart Lung 2015;44:521–7.

Pain Management in the Individual with Serious Illness and Comorbid Substance Use Disorder

CrossMark

Anne F. Walsh, ANP-BC, CWOCN, ACHPN[a], Kathleen Broglio, DNP, ANP-BC, ACHPN, CPE, FPCN[b],*

KEYWORDS

- Advanced disease • Drug addiction • Hospice • Pain management • Palliative care
- Serious illness • Substance use disorder

KEY POINTS

- Pain is prevalent in individuals with serious illness and comorbid substance use disorder and requires a comprehensive assessment and treatment plan.
- A comprehensive pain assessment includes risk assessment for misuse of opioid medications.
- "Universal precautions" should be used when designing a pain management treatment protocol for all individuals.
- Pain management in individuals with serious illness and comorbid substance use disorder requires a unified interdisciplinary team approach.

Case study

John is a 45-year-old man with metastatic non–small cell lung cancer with extensive bony metastases. Before the diagnosis, he experienced lower back pain and his primary medical team prescribed him immediate-release opioids and referred him for further workup. Because of insurance issues, he delayed further workup and began obtaining analgesic medications from friends. As his pain worsened, he started to use heroin to control the pain.

Although he is now receiving treatment, including radiotherapy to the spinal bony metastases, he has continued pain. He has had intolerances or lack of efficacy to multiple opioids, and has refused to take extended-release opioids stating that they do not work. His pain is now being treated with hydromorphone 8 to 16 mg orally every 3 hours as needed for pain and at times, he is using more than 200 mg daily. He is followed weekly in the palliative care clinic and each time he is seen he is out of medications. During a recent hospitalization, there was a concern that he was injecting the oral medications and tampering with the patient-controlled analgesia machine.

Disclosures: No disclosures (A.F. Walsh); Consulting fees – Purdue Pharmaceuticals, Emmi Solutions; speaker's bureau Genentech, Mallinkrodt; Royalties – UpToDate (K. Broglio).

[a] Visiting Nurse Service of New York, Hospice and Palliative Care, 1250 Broadway, 7th Floor, New York, NY 10001, USA; [b] Section of Palliative Medicine, Dartmouth Hitchcock Medical Center, 1 Medical Center Drive, Lebanon, NH 03756, USA
* Corresponding author.
E-mail address: kathleen.broglio@me.com

INTRODUCTION

Individuals with serious illnesses including cancer often have unmanaged pain.[1,2] In a systematic review of 40 years of cancer treatment, 24% to 60% of those undergoing treatment, 58% to 69% of those with advanced cancer and 33% of cancer survivors experienced pain.[3] According to Laroche and colleagues,[4] pain is a common reason for persons with drug addiction to seek medical care. People with a history of substance use disorder (SUD) face a risk of undertreated pain often due to clinician biases and regulatory fears.[2,4,5] Nurses must possess the knowledge and skills to ensure appropriate and safe pain management in this population.

PREVALENCE OF SUBSTANCE USE DISORDER

According to the Substance Abuse and Mental Health Services Administration (SAMHSA) national survey data on drug use and health, an estimated 24.6 million adults (9.4% of US population 12 years old or older) used illicit drugs in 2013.[6] Although marijuana has continued to be the most commonly used drug, the nonmedical use of pain relievers (opioids) is the second most commonly misused class of medications.[6] Results from the SAMHSA survey also showed that nearly 1 (18.5%) in 5 adults 18 years old or older have a mental illness.[6] Drug abuse is more prevalent in those with mood disorders or anxiety.[7–9] With the increased use of opioids for chronic pain, opioid prescriptions increased from approximately 76 million in 1991 to almost 207 million in 2013.[10] With this increase in opioid availability, there has been an increase in unintentional deaths, more than quadrupling since 1999.[10] According to the US Centers for Disease Control and Prevention (CDC), a total of 47,055 drug overdose deaths occurred in the United States in 2014.[11] Opioids and heroin were responsible for 28,647 (61%) of these drug overdose deaths.[11]

Earlier studies have reported less prevalence of substance abuse in individuals with serious illnesses.[12] These estimates may not be adequate because of underreporting or access to care barriers for those with SUDs.[12] Chesher and colleagues[13] found that individuals entering treatment facilities for SUD have a higher incidence of chronic illnesses, such as asthma and hypertension, in addition to mental illnesses, and are more likely to be using tobacco, leading to a higher incidence of morbidity and mortality. A recent study on risk stratification for those with cancer pain found that the number of those with SUD risk factors were similar to those in the chronic pain population.[14] Although there are limited recent data available on the prevalence of SUD in those with serious illnesses, it likely can be extrapolated from the studies of the general population.[15,16] Until more studies are conducted that adequately reflect the true prevalence of SUD in this population, safeguards should be in place to address the potential for substance misuse.[12]

SCOPE OF PROBLEM IN HOSPICE AND PALLIATIVE CARE

Data about the scope of the problem in hospice and palliative care are limited. Pancari and Baird[17] point out the risks for opioid misuse and diversion when patients are receiving home hospice services where there may be limited oversight and where large quantities of opioids may be delivered to the home to manage uncontrolled symptoms. Risks may be higher in the home population than previously reported, as more than 70% of prescription drugs that are diverted or otherwise misused are by family and friends.[6] Blackhall and colleagues[1] found that training policies for handling patient and family substance abuse and diversion issues within hospices were lacking in Virginia. Most palliative care programs surveyed did not have policies in place for addressing substance abuse or diversion issues and were not consistently screening patients for the risk of SUD.[16] In a recent survey, fewer than 50% of palliative medicine fellows had received adequate training in addiction and in managing opioid misuse, and most did not feel prepared to treat pain in this population.[18] Thus, to effectively manage this problem, palliative and hospice programs must develop systemwide policies and provide training for providers to decrease the risk for harm from opioid diversion and substance misuse.

CLARIFYING TERMINOLOGY

Lack of standardized terminology and appropriate use among health care providers complicates the problem. The use of inappropriate terminology and labeling of individuals with possible SUDs hinders appropriate care. In addition, some of the defining elements of SUD, such as "social impairment" may not be applicable to the individual with a serious illness due to declining functional status from disease progression.[12] Health care providers must exercise care when using these terms, as careless use of the word "addiction" may create biases that limit appropriate treatment for the individual in future encounters. For the purpose of this discussion, a brief description of the commonly used terms follows.

Substance use disorder, the official term of the American Psychiatric Association, is the use of alcohol and/or other substances for nonmedical purposes that can exist on a continuum from mild to severe.[19,20] *Physical dependence* is an altered physiologic state caused by repeated administration of certain drug classes that if stopped abruptly or if an antagonistic medication is administered, could lead to withdrawal symptoms[19,21]; this does not necessarily constitute addiction. Physical dependence can occur with medications such as steroids, antidepressants, or beta-blockers, where cessation of the medication can cause withdrawal symptoms. On the other hand, *tolerance* is a state of adaptation in which, after repeated administration of a drug, the dose produces a decreased effect over time requiring larger doses to obtain the same effect. It also refers to decreased side effects, such as nausea from pain medications, as tolerance develops.[19,21] *Addiction* is a complex, neurobiological disease in which there is compulsive use of a substance, impaired control over its use, craving for the substance, and the continued use despite the risk for harm.[19,22] It is important to note this is a complex phenomenon and is not just dependent on environmental circumstances. *Pseudoaddiction* is a term used when inadequately treated pain leads to behaviors that resemble addiction, but these behaviors resolve with improved pain management.[23] However, this term is based on clinical case studies versus empirical evidence,[24] so further research is necessary to fully describe the signs and symptoms and the differentiation between this phenomenon and addiction (**Box 1**).[25]

In clinical care, the concept of "aberrant drug-related behavior" has developed into a model that can guide clinicians. These behaviors may be representative of addiction issues or could be related to inadequate analgesia or psychological distress.[12] Aberrant drug-taking behaviors can range from mildly aberrant to more highly aberrant behaviors. Mildly aberrant behaviors, such as hoarding medications, borrowing from family and friends, and requests for specific medications, may be representative of unrelieved pain or patient distress.[12] Whereas behaviors such as prescription forgery, obtaining medications from nonmedical sources, selling medications, or crushing opioids for injection or nasal use are more highly aberrant behaviors that warrant immediate intervention.[2,12] If individuals are engaged in these behaviors, further evaluation is warranted (**Box 2**).

Box 1
Standardized terminology

Substance use disorder
- Use of alcohol and or other substances for nonmedical purposes and can range on a continuum from mild to severe.

Addiction: Primary, chronic neurobiological disease with genetic, psychosocial, and environmental factors influencing its development and manifestation
- Characterized by behaviors that include 1 or more of the following: impaired control over drug use, compulsive use, continued use despite harm, and craving

Physical Dependence: State of adaptation that is manifested by a drug class
- Syndrome that can be produced by abrupt cessation, rapid dose reduction, decreasing blood levels of drug and/or administration of an antagonist

Tolerance: State of adaptation in which the exposure to a drug induces changes that result in a diminution of one or more of the drug's effects over time
- Ex: decreases the opioid's side effects such as nausea, pruritus, and respiratory depression
- May decrease the analgesic's ability to reduce pain at the current dose

Pseudoaddiction
- Inadequately treated pain leads to behaviors that resemble addiction, but these behaviors resolve with improved pain management

Data from Refs.[19,20,23]

SUBSTANCE USE DISORDER ON A CONTINUUM

SUD can be viewed as occurring along a continuum. The individual may have an active SUD, may be in a methadone or buprenorphine maintenance recovery program, or may have a remote history of alcohol or drug abuse and not be participating in a maintenance program or support group. Individuals with a remote history of alcohol or drug abuse may fear relapse when being treated with opioids for pain.[2] Research is lacking about the risk for reactivating a substance abuse episode or dependency in those with

---

Box 2
Behaviors more likely related to drug aberrancy

- Prescription forgery
- Illicit drug abuse
- Crushing analgesics for injection or insufflation
- Prescription drug sales
- Multiple dose escalations without notifying provider
- Stealing other's drugs
- Obtaining prescription drugs from nonmedical sources
- Recurrent prescription losses

Data from Kirsh KL, Compton P, Egan-City K, et al. Caring for the patient with substance use disorder at the end of life. In: Ferrell BR, Coyle N, editors. Textbook of palliative nursing. New York: Oxford University Press; 2015. p. 650–60; and Price JR, Hawkins AD, Passik SD. Opioid therapy: managing risks of abuse, addiction, and diversion. In: Cherny NI, Fallon MT, Kaasa S, et al, editors. Oxford textbook of palliative medicine. 5th edition. Oxford (United Kingdom): Oxford University Press; 2015. p. 560–6.

a previous substance abuse history.[12] Much of the research on SUD and pain management focused on individuals with chronic noncancer pain, with little research on those with advanced illnesses, SUD, and pain.[2,15] Therefore, until further research is conducted in this population, one can extrapolate the findings from the current research to provide effective and safe pain management.

UNIVERSAL PRECAUTIONS

Although it is imperative to treat the individual's pain, which may require opioid therapy, it is also critical to have safeguards against opioid misuse in place.[1,2,5,12,16] When treating individuals with chronic pain with opioid therapy, the use of a "universal precautions" approach has been recommended.[26] With this approach, all patients would be treated as if they are at risk for addiction. This is an effective strategy because clinicians may not always identify individuals who are at risk for abusing opioids. A universal precautions approach also reduces the stigma associated with labeling an individual as at-risk and also can protect the practitioner who again may not perceive that there is a potential for a substance use problem with the individual.[22] The elements for universal precautions in opioid prescribing include the following: a comprehensive pain assessment and risk assessment for misuse; differential diagnosis for the pain; informed consent; clear documentation of the treatment plan, decision making, and goals for opioid therapy; ongoing reassessment of analgesia effects; and the use of urine drug screening as needed.[26] Although the intent of this approach was for individuals with chronic pain, it should be a consideration for care in those with serious illness and pain who require opioid therapy.

PAIN ASSESSMENT

A comprehensive pain assessment is the critical first step for effective pain management. The assessment should include the pain location(s), duration, onset, and characteristics to identify nociceptive versus neuropathic pain; aggravating factors, such as wound care or activity; relieving factors, such as heat/ice or rest; other past successful treatments both pharmacologic and nonpharmacologic; associated symptoms, such as depression, anxiety, or insomnia; adverse side effects from analgesics, such as sedation, nausea, and constipation; and realistic pain management goals.[27,28] The comprehensive pain assessment also should include an assessment for the risk of opioid misuse if opioids may be a consideration for treatment. The risk assessment should include specific drug use history (important to avoid withdrawal or drug interactions), comorbid psychiatric conditions, history of preadolescent sexual abuse, smoking/alcohol use history, family history of SUD, and details of the home environment.[27] To establish rapport, the assessment may start with questions about smoking and alcohol use history, explaining that these questions are asked of all individuals requiring pain management and that the information is needed to develop a safe, effective treatment plan. For those in recovery programs, permission to contact the methadone or buprenorphine maintenance program is obtained, as this is necessary for collaboration.[2,22]

Opioid risk assessment or evaluation tools can be used with individuals with pain and serious illness. However, at the time of this writing, the tools have been validated only in those patients with chronic nonmalignant pain. These tools can be used as part of the decision-making process for opioid prescribing. A recent study in a cancer population evaluated the use of the Screener and Opioid Assessment for Patients in Pain Short Form (SOAPP-SF), but the study was limited because of lack of comparison with other tools.[14] Other commonly used tools include the Opioid Risk Tool (ORT),[29] the

Screener and Opioid Assessment for Patients in Pain–Revised (SOAPP-R),[30] and the Diagnosis, Intractability, Risk, Efficacy Score (DIRES) tool.[31] The CAGE (cutting down, annoyance by criticism, guilty feeling, eye opener) is an easy-to-administer, validated tool to screen for alcoholism[32] and has been adapted to include screening for drug abuse (CAGE-AID)[33] (**Table 1**). Although the previously mentioned tools are used to assess for substance abuse risk, all have their limitations.[34,35] The tool selection will depend on the clinical setting and its ease of implementation. The one caveat is that these tools do not assess for the risk of diversion by family or friends, so a thorough family and social history is part of the risk assessment process.

Even if the results of the opioid risk evaluation tool show the individual has a low-risk score, the decision to use opioids should not be made solely on this one criterion. If the history and the risk score indicate that the patient is at a high risk for misusing opioids, or the individual has an active SUD or major untreated mental illness, treatment should be in conjunction with a pain or addiction specialist.[26] In many settings, these specialists may not be readily available, thus the use of universal precautions with a multidisciplinary approach is even more essential.

Tools to monitor for adherence to therapy for those already being treated with opioids include the Current Opioid Misuse Measure (COMM),[36] and the Pain Assessment Documentation Tool (PADT).[37] The PADT is a user-friendly tool that incorporates important components of the pain assessment documentation that include analgesia efficacy, activities of daily living, adverse effects of medications, and signs of aberrant behavior (the 4 A's).[37] Clinicians often include assessment of the patient's "affect or

Table 1
Opioid risk assessment tools

Opioid Risk Assessment Tools[a]	Key Points	Sample Forms
Assess risk for opioid abuse before starting chronic opioid therapy		
Diagnosis, Intractability, Risk, Efficacy (DIRE)	7 items patient interview	http://integratedcare-nw.org/DIRE_score.pdf
Opioid Risk Tool (ORT)	5 items self-administer	http://www.partnersagainstpain.com/printouts/Opioid_Risk_Tool.pdf
Screener and Opioid Assessment for Patients with Pain–Revised (SOAPP-R)	24 items self-administer	http://nationalpaincentre.mcmaster.ca/documents/soapp_r_sample_watermark.pdf
CAGE- AID (cutting down, annoyance by criticism, guilty feeling, eye opener adapted to include drugs)	4 items patient interview Adapted from CAGE tool for alcoholism	https://www.mhn.com/static/pdfs/CAGE-AID.pdf
Ongoing assessment tools for patients on opioid therapy		
Current Opioid Misuse Measure (COMM)	17 items self-administer	http://www.etsu.edu/com/cme/documents/kptt2012/7-COMM_Final_SAMPLE.pdf
Pain Assessment and Documentation Tool (PADT)	41 items (chart note documentation)	http://www.prescriberesponsibly.com/sites/default/files/pdf/pain/PADT.pdf

[a] This is only a sample list of a few tools that the authors find useful. Information on more tools is available at Opioid Risk http://www.opioidrisk.com/node/775 (site last updated February 17, 2016).

mood," a fifth "A," which although not part of the original tool, is a key component in reassessment,[5] as it may alert the practitioner for the need for further assessment for mood disorders that can inhibit effective pain management. Although improvements in activities of daily living may not be a feasible measure for the individual with progressive serious illness, it is a good indicator if the medications are helping with function in those who have functional limitations due to pain.

MANAGEMENT STRATEGIES

Multiple pain management guidelines are available to assist clinicians caring for individuals with pain. Guidelines and recommendations for safe prescribing of opioids can be extrapolated for use in those with serious illness.[27,38–41] The use of a multimodal analgesia model (using medications from different drug classes) is a key component to effective pain management in acute pain[40] and is a consideration for use in cancer-related pain.[42] The World Health Organization (WHO) analgesic ladder is a widely used stepwise multimodal pain management algorithm, which has been revised to include interventional therapies as options for pain management.[43] The National Comprehensive Cancer Network (NCCN) provides comprehensive cancer pain management guidelines that have been updated to include assessment for risk of substance abuse and recommendations for safe opioid prescribing.[44] Due to the increasing concern about prescription drug abuse, the Food and Drug Administration (FDA) mandated the availability of education about the use of extended-release and long-acting opioids in an effort to improve knowledge about the prescribing of these medications, and to decrease the risk of abuse and diversion.[45] The Risk Evaluation Mitigation Strategy (REMS) for opioid education includes significant material on risk assessment and management of opioid therapy[45] and is recommended for all prescribers treating pain. A full discussion of specific recommendations for pain management is beyond the scope of this article, but the essential components are briefly discussed here.

Informed Consent and Treatment Agreements

Multiple experts and organizations have recommended the use of patient prescriber treatment agreements before the initiation of opioid therapy.[26,39,40,46] Agreements can be useful not only to outline the responsibilities of the patient and the prescriber, but also to include education about the safe use and disposal of opioids and the risks and benefits associated with opioid therapy.[47] Ultimately the goal is to reduce the risks of aberrant drug-taking behavior.[12] However, there is limited evidence that the use of these agreements decreases the risk of opioid misuse.[39–41,46] Literature is sparse about the use of treatment agreements when prescribing opioids in the setting of serious illness, but there has been increased use among palliative care providers in the outpatient clinical setting (American Academy Hospice Palliative Medicine Community Blogs, personal communications, 2016). Treatment agreements should be easy to read and at a level consistent with the health literacy of the patient population. Examples of treatment agreements are available for download[48] and the included example can be adapted for use (**Fig. 1**).

Urine Drug Testing

Urine drug testing (UDT) is an objective measure to determine if the individual is taking what is being prescribed, is using illicit drugs, or is taking prescription medications that have not been prescribed. Although there is not extensive evidence for the use of UDT to prevent misuse, obtaining a UDT before initiating opioid therapy and randomly

SAMPLE
Patient Provider Informed Consent and Treatment Agreement
DATE: _____/_____/_____   MR# _____

I _____ agree to the following conditions:
- ☐ I understand I have a pain condition that may be helped with the use of an opioid.
- ☐ I will obtain prescriptions for opioids only from my treating clinician. If I am prescribed other controlled substances such as benzodiazepines (i.e.; lorazepam, alprazolam) or sleep aides (i.e. zolpidem) from another health care provider, I will provide this information to my treating clinician
- ☐ I will have prescriptions filled at only one pharmacy
  Pharmacy Name:_____ Telephone Number:_____
- ☐ I understand that prescriptions will be given only during the scheduled appointments.
- ☐ I will take medications only as prescribed and will promptly notify my treating clinician if I am not taking medications as prescribed
- ☐ I agree to random urine or blood tests
- ☐ I agree to initial and follow up psychological evaluation if recommended by my health care provider
- ☐ I will meet regularly with my treating clinician to assess my response to treatment
- ☐ Lost, misplaced, or stolen prescriptions and/or substances will not be replaced.
- ☐ I understand that prescriptions will not be replaced if I do not have them filled within 30 days of their issue.
- ☐ Refill prescriptions will not be provided other than at the scheduled visits
- ☐ I agree not to use illicit drugs (i.e.; heroin, cocaine) or medications that are not prescribed to me
- ☐ I will not share or sell my medications
- ☐ I will keep my medications in a secure place, preferable a locked box
- ☐ Side effects to opioids such as nausea, constipation, and increased sedation and the use of medications to counteract these side effects have been explained to me.
- ☐ Long-term side effects of opioids, which may include decreases in testosterone level (men), or cessation of menstrual cycle (women) have been explained to me.
- ☐ I understand that I may be tapered off the opioids for any of the following reasons:
  - ✓ I deviate from the above guidelines
  - ✓ The substance(s) are not effective
  - ✓ If illegal drugs are found in my urine
  - ✓ If there is evidence of the misuse of medications
  - ✓ Non-compliance with clinical pain team medical recommendations
  - ✓ Changes of treatment plan based on Health Care Provider reassessment
- ☐ Risks of dependence and addiction have been discussed with me
- ☐ I understand the contents of this agreement and I consent to treatment with an opioid.

Patient's Name	_____	Patient's Signature	_____
Clinician Name	_____	Clinician Signature	_____
Witness' Name	_____	Witness' Signature	_____

Fig. 1. Sample informed consent and patient-prescriber agreement. (*Adapted from* Walsh AF, Broglio K. Pain management in advanced illness and comorbid substance use disorder. J Hosp Palliat Nurs 2010;12(1):12; with permission.)

during chronic opioid therapy is strongly recommended.[39–41,46,49] Point of care "dipstick" urine tests are easily performed in the office setting; however, this test will evaluate only "classes" of medications, but not specific medications, thus is not recommended for those on chronic opioid therapy.[49] Additionally if the individual is taking semisynthetic opioids, such as fentanyl or oxycodone, the dipstick test may not identify opioids in the urine. Gas chromatography/mass spectrometry UDT is the recommended test for those on chronic opioid therapy. This test will identify the specific substances (eg, hydromorphone vs oxycodone) and metabolites of opioids (ie, oxymorphone, noroxycodone) present in the urine.[49] No consensus exists about the frequency of testing, but more frequent testing may be necessary for those who are at a high risk for substance abuse or for those who are actively abusing substances.[49] It is important to understand the laboratory's capability and how to interpret the test results. For those patients who are homebound, challenges may exist in obtaining UDTs. Because gas chromatography/mass spectrometry UDT can be expensive, hospice programs will need to consider the feasibility of use, because the costs will be absorbed by the hospice program.

When the results of the urine drug screen are inconsistent with prescribed therapy, the course of action may be dictated by the policies of the practice or by the established treatment agreement. In the case of illicit drug use, such as heroin or cocaine, the decision may be to discontinue opioid therapy and refer the individual to a treatment program. When the prescribed medication is not in the urine, it is important to discuss this with the individual, as reasons may include skipping doses, running out of medications, or diversion of the opioid. The decision to continue therapy will be dependent on the assessment and the goals of care. For someone approaching the end of life, practitioners may decide to continue opioid therapy even in cases in which individuals are abusing illicit drugs. In these cases, clinicians may use strategies for harm reduction, such as using transdermal opioid therapies and limiting the use of breakthrough opioid medications and/or increasing the use of nonopioid adjuvant medications and nonpharmacological pain interventions.

Prescription Monitoring Programs and Electronic Prescribing

The use of prescription drug monitoring programs (PDMP or PMP) is another recommended strategy to decrease misuse or diversion of opioids.[39,50] As of December 2014, 49 states and 1 US territory had operational PDMP programs.[51] The programs are state specific and differ in accessibility and functionality. Early data from the use of PDMPs indicate that the use of these programs may decrease abuse or misuse.[52] However, it is difficult to check the status in neighboring states without registering for that state-specific program. In certain states, the use of the PDMP is mandatory before prescribing opioids; early data showed changes in prescribing patterns in these states.[53] Hospice prescribers may be exempt from checking PDMPs before prescribing opioids at this time,[54] but each clinician should check their state's regulations. Despite some of the challenges, the use of PDMPs may be useful in the palliative care and hospice setting to track prescriptions, especially if multiple providers are treating the individual. The use of electronic prescribing of opioids may improve not only opioid tracking, but may also decrease the risk of prescription forgery.[55,56] Electronic prescribing of opioids may be mandated in certain states[57] and its use is likely to increase over time.

Opioid Selection

Opioid therapy decisions are often based on the prescriber's clinical comfort level and increasingly are dictated by insurance coverage. Mu-agonist opioids can trigger the "reward" system producing euphoria through binding to GABAergic interneurons, which inhibit dopamine production.[22] For those with histories of substance abuse, the activation of this reward system can trigger the craving and thus possibly the misuse of opioids.[22] Immediate-release opioids (such as oxycodone/acetaminophen, hydromorphone) have a faster onset and increase of blood levels, which can trigger the "reward" system.[22] Although no robust evidence exists about the superior efficacy of extended-release opioids versus short-acting opioids to manage pain and decrease misuse, extended-release opioids may produce longer periods of stable analgesia, improve sleep, and improve physical function.[58] And more importantly for those with histories of substance abuse or those at risk for misuse, the use of an extended-release opioid (eg, morphine extended release, transdermal fentanyl) or a long-acting formulation (eg, methadone) decreases the "reward" or the "likeability" component of the medication's effect.[22]

Due to the escalation of prescription drug abuse, the FDA has provided guidance to the industry for future opioid development to ensure that the opioids are more difficult to tamper with and have a reduced likeability.[59] New formulations of extended-release opioids incorporate either physical barrier to prevent crushing or contain either antagonists or irritants if the tablet is altered and ingested.[58,60] The emergence of formulations that are abuse-deterrent or tamper-resistant may help in minimizing the abuse of opioids, but may be cost prohibitive for use in the hospice and palliative care settings because, at the time of this writing, these medications are not yet available as generic formulations.

DESIGNING A SAFE TREATMENT PLAN

In addition to the universal precautions strategies discussed previously, other measures can be undertaken to minimize opioid abuse risk and avoid diversion. Complete documentation of the plan of care that can be easily accessed by all team members is a critical aspect to decrease the potential for abuse and harm.[22] As noted previously, the use of extended-release or long-acting opioids, such as methadone, is recommended.[22] Specific instructions on the time of day of medication administration (ie, 800 AM, 400 PM) versus every 8-hours dosing may be more effective to minimize confusion about administration.[22] In patients with serious illness who may experience breakthrough pain and require the use of immediate-release opioids, it may be necessary to put safeguards, such as making the medication time contingent or related to a painful activity versus relying only on the pain severity, as an indicator for use.[22]

When considering the use of immediate-release opioids, one should avoid prescribing high street-value medications to avert diversion. These medications may vary according to the geographic location. For example, oxycodone 30-mg tablets have a high street value in the New York City region. Individuals who require repeated dose escalations should be reassessed for potential reasons for the inefficacy of the opioid or the possibility of diversion or misuse.[22,26] The use of nonopioid adjuvants as part of the pain management plan is an important component, as escalating doses of opioids may not always adequately address the pain.[22,47]

For patients in pain who are enrolled in methadone or buprenorphine maintenance programs, close collaboration with the team at the facility is essential. The maintenance dose will likely not be sufficient to manage the pain if the disease process that is causing the pain is progressive. The program may continue the maintenance dose and another opioid used for pain or additional methadone may be added in divided doses prescribed by the clinician.[22]

Frequent follow-up visits to assess for appropriate use of prescribed medications, including urine toxicology screens, are an important component of care.[22] If the patient is at home and seen by a home palliative care or hospice agency, frequent visits by members of the team should be scheduled.[47] It is preferable to have one prescriber and one pharmacy,[22,47] but in the cases in which there is cross-coverage, a detailed plan should be agreed on and documented to ensure consistency among providers. A limited supply of opioids should be prescribed and dispensed, especially for high-risk patients.[22,27,47] In cases of those individuals at very high risk for opioid misuse, consideration can be given to daily visits by members of the team and for using fentanyl patches in the home or clinical setting, without dispensing a supply of oral pain medications.[22] When feasible, family and/or friends should be involved in the care to help ensure compliance and ensure appropriate and safe pain management.[2,12] Finally, it is important to ensure safety in the home setting by keeping medications safely secured, such as in lockboxes, to prevent diversion or theft.[22,47] Individuals and families should be educated on measures to take in the event of adverse events, such as oversedation secondary to opioids.[61] Naloxone in intramuscular and intranasal forms was available in 37 states as of July 2015 for laypersons so that family/friends have the ability to help prevent death from an accidental overdose.[62] Education can include training caregivers to administer naloxone in the event of an overdose.[62] Patient education should also include safe disposal of medications or the use of Drug Enforcement Agency (DEA) take-back programs.[63,64] In the hospice setting, policies should be in place for proper medication disposal after a patient dies or when there is a rotation to another opioid before the previous opioid supply is finished.

Due to the high probability of comorbid mental illness in the patient with SUD, an interdisciplinary approach is essential. The team members may include physicians, physician assistants, nurse practitioners, a psychiatrist, psychologist, an addiction specialist, registered nurses, social workers, and spiritual care counselors.[12,47] For those with chronic pain without a life-limiting illness, participation in counseling or programs, such as Narcotics Anonymous, should be an expectation.[22] Although this may not be practical for the individual with a serious illness, in those cases in which the individual is well enough to attend appointments and participate in activities of daily living, this may be a consideration.

SPECIAL CONSIDERATIONS IN THE ACUTE CARE OR INPATIENT HOSPICE SETTING

In the inpatient setting or at times at home, patients may be treated for pain through intravenous routes when the pain is severe. In these settings, patient-controlled analgesia (PCA) may provide pain benefit through small incremental dosing, which is preferable to intermittent clinician bolus dosing, which may trigger the reward system. The PCA also allows the individual some control over the bolus dosing and may reduce the perception that there is "drug-seeking," which can occur when the patient is receiving intermittent or as-needed doses of medications administered by clinicians.[22] Safeguards should be in place to ensure appropriate monitoring of the patient to minimize untoward side effects. Patient education should include instructions that only the patient should administer bolus dosing.[65] Lockboxes or methods of securing the medication also should be used to minimize the risk of tampering with the medication in the PCA. For individuals who are actively abusing drugs, extra precautions may be necessary for those who have intravenous access to prevent use of illicit substances via this route. In certain cases, visitor restriction or searching of patient's belongings may be necessary to prevent substance abuse in the inpatient setting.[12]

SUMMARY

Individuals with comorbid SUD who are experiencing pain due to a serious illness have a right to effective pain management. A comprehensive pain and opioid risk assessment, the use of multimodal analgesia, and communication among all providers are essential components of a safe treatment plan. An effective pain treatment plan often includes opioids when the pain is severe and cannot be controlled with nonopioid medications. It cannot be stressed enough that all clinicians should strive to minimize biases and provide treatment in a competent, compassionate manner.

REFERENCES

1. Blackhall LJ, Alfson ED, Barclay JS. Screening for substance abuse and diversion in virginia hospices. J Palliat Med 2013;16(3):237–42.
2. Kirsh KL, Compton P, Egan-City K, et al. Caring for the patient with substance use disorder at the end of life. In: Ferrell BR, Coyle N, Paice J, editors. Oxford textbook of palliative nursing. 4th edition. New York: Oxford University Press; 2015. p. 650–60.
3. van den Beuken-van Everdingen MH, de Rijke JM, Kessels AG, et al. Prevalence of pain in patients with cancer: a systematic review of the past 40 years. Ann Oncol 2007;18(9):1437–49.
4. Laroche F, Rostaing S, Aubrun F, et al. Pain management in heroin and cocaine users. Joint Bone Spine 2012;79(5):446–50.
5. Oliver J, Coggins C, Compton P, et al. American Society for Pain Management nursing position statement: pain management in patients with substance use disorders. Pain Manag Nurs 2012;13(3):169–83.
6. Substance Abuse and Mental Health Services Administration. Results from the 2013 national survey on drug use and health: summary of national findings. Rockville (MD): Substance Abuse and Mental Health Services Administration; 2014. p. 2014.
7. National Institute of Drug Abuse. Comorbidity: addiction and other mental illnesses. U. S. Department of Health and Human Services; 2008. Available at: http://www.drugabuse.gov/publications/comorbidity-addiction-other-mental-illnesses/why-do-drug-use-disorders-often-co-occur-other-mental-illnesses.
8. Gros DF, Milanak ME, Brady KT, et al. Frequency and severity of comorbid mood and anxiety disorders in prescription opioid dependence. Am J Addict 2013; 22(3):261–5.
9. Probst DR, Wells-Di Gregorio S, Marks DR. Suffering compounded: the relationship between abuse history and distress in five palliative care domains. J Palliat Med 2013;16(10):1242–8.
10. National Institute of Drug Abuse. Prescription opioid and heroin abuse. House Committee on Energy and Commerce Subcommittee on Oversight and Investigations. National Institute of Health; 2014. Available at: https://www.drugabuse.gov/about-nida/legislative-activities/testimony-to-congress/2015/prescription-opioid-heroin-abuse.
11. Rudd RA, Aleshire A, Zibbell JE, et al. Increases in drug and opioid overdose deaths—United States, 2000-2014. US DHHS/CDC. MMWR Morb Mortal Wkly Rep 2016;64(50 & 51):1378–82.
12. Price JRHA, Passik SD. Opioid therapy: managing risks of abuse, addiction, and diversion. In: Cherny NI, Fallon M, Kaasa S, et al, editors. Oxford textbook of palliative medicine. 5th edition. Oxford (United Kingdom): Oxford University Press; 2015. p. 560–6.
13. Chesher NJ, Bousman CA, Gale M, et al. Chronic illness histories of adults entering treatment for co-occurring substance abuse and other mental health disorders. Am J Addict 2012;21(1):1–4.
14. Koyyalagunta D, Bruera E, Aigner C, et al. Risk stratification of opioid misuse among patients with cancer pain using the SOAPP-R. Pain Med 2013;14(5): 667–75.
15. Reisfield GM, Paulian GD, Wilson GR. Substance use disorders in the palliative care patient #127. J Palliat Med 2009;12(5):475–6.

16. Tan PD, Barclay JS, Blackhall LJ. Do palliative care clinics screen for substance abuse and diversion? Results of a national survey. J Palliat Med 2015;18(9): 752–7.

17. Pancari J, Baird C. Managing prescription drug diversion risks: caring for individuals at home. J Addict Nurs 2014;25(3):114–21.

18. Childers JW, Arnold RM. "I feel uncomfortable 'calling a patient out'": educational needs of palliative medicine fellows in managing opioid misuse. J Pain Symptom Manage 2012;43(2):253–60.

19. Wilford BB. Appendix 1: ASAM addiction terminology. In: Ries RK, Fiellin DA, Miller SC, et al, editors. The ASAM principles of addiction medicine. 5th edition. Philadelphia: Wolters Kluwer; 2014.

20. American Psychiatric Association. Diagnostic and statistical manual of mental disorders: DSM-5. Washington, DC: American Psychiatric Association; 2013.

21. Zajicek A, Karan LD. Pharmacokinetics and pharmacodynamic principles. In: Herron AJ, Brennan TK, editors. The ASAM essentials of addiction medicine. 2nd edition. Philadelphia: Wolters Kluwer; 2015. p. 41–6.

22. Savage SR. Opioid therapy for pain. In: Ries RK, Fiellin DA, Miller SC, et al, editors. The ASAM principles of addiction medicine. 5th edition. Philadelphia: Wolters Kluwer; 2014. p. 1500–29.

23. Weissman DE, Haddox JD. Opioid pseudoaddiction–an iatrogenic syndrome. Pain 1989;36(3):363–6.

24. Greene MS, Chambers RA. Pseudoaddiction: fact or fiction? An investigation of the medical literature. Curr Addict Rep 2015;2(4):310–7.

25. Passik SD, Kirsh KL, Webster L. Pseudoaddiction revisited: a commentary on clinical and historical considerations. Pain Manag 2011;1(3):239–48.

26. Gourlay DL, Heit HA. Universal precautions revisited: managing the inherited pain patient. Pain Med 2009;10(Suppl 2):S115–23.

27. Broglio K, Cole BE. Prescribing opioids in primary care: avoiding perils and pitfalls. Nurse Pract 2014;39(6):30–7 [quiz: 37–8].

28. McCaffery M, Herr K, Pasero C. Assessment tools. In: Pasero C, McCaffery M, editors. Pain assessment and pharmacologic management. St Louis (MO): Mosby Elsevier; 2011. p. 49–142.

29. Webster LR, Webster RM. Predicting aberrant behaviors in opioid-treated patients: preliminary validation of the opioid risk tool. Pain Med 2005;6(6):432–42.

30. Butler SF, Fernandez K, Benoit C, et al. Validation of the revised screener and opioid assessment for patients with pain (SOAPP-R). J Pain 2008;9(4):360–72.

31. Belgrade MJ, Schamber CD, Lindgren BR. The dire score: predicting outcomes of opioid prescribing for chronic pain. J Pain 2006;7(9):671–81.

32. Dhalla S, Kopec JA. The CAGE questionnaire for alcohol misuse: a review of reliability and validity studies. Clin Invest Med 2007;30(1):33–41.

33. Brown RL, Rounds LA. Conjoint screening questionnaires for alcohol and other drug abuse: criterion validity in a primary care practice. Wis Med J 1995;94(3): 135–40.

34. Sehgal N, Manchikanti L, Smith HS. Prescription opioid abuse in chronic pain: a review of opioid abuse predictors and strategies to curb opioid abuse. Pain Physician 2012;15(3 Suppl):ES67–92.

35. Solanki DR, Koyyalagunta D, Shah RV, et al. Monitoring opioid adherence in chronic pain patients: assessment of risk of substance misuse. Pain Physician 2011;14(2):E119–31.

36. Butler SF, Budman SH, Fernandez KC, et al. Development and validation of the current opioid misuse measure. Pain 2007;130(1–2):144–56.

37. Passik SD, Kirsh KL, Whitcomb L, et al. A new tool to assess and document pain outcomes in chronic pain patients receiving opioid therapy. Clin Ther 2004;26(4): 552–61.

38. Manchikanti L, Abdi S, Atluri S, et al. American Society of Interventional Pain Physicians (ASIPP) guidelines for responsible opioid prescribing in chronic non-cancer pain: part I–evidence assessment. Pain Physician 2012;15(3 Suppl): S1–65.

39. Manchikanti L, Abdi S, Atluri S, et al. American Society of Interventional Pain Physicians (ASIPP) guidelines for responsible opioid prescribing in chronic non-cancer pain: Part 2–guidance. Pain Physician 2012;15(3 Suppl):S67–116.

40. Chou R, Fanciullo GJ, Fine PG, et al. Clinical guidelines for the use of chronic opioid therapy in chronic noncancer pain. J Pain 2009;10(2):113–30.

41. Nuckols TK, Anderson L, Popescu I, et al. Opioid prescribing: a systematic review and critical appraisal of guidelines for chronic pain. Ann Intern Med 2014; 160(1):38–47.

42. Afsharimani B, Kindl K, Good P, et al. Pharmacological options for the management of refractory cancer pain—what is the evidence? Support Care Cancer 2015;23(5):1473–81.

43. Vargas-Schaffer G. Is the WHO analgesic ladder still valid? Twenty-four years of experience. Can Fam Physician 2010;56(6):514–7, e202-5.

44. National Comprehensive Cancer Network. Clinical practice guidelines in oncology (NCCN guidelines); adult cancer pain. National Comprehensive Cancer Network; 2015. Available at: https://www.nccn.org/store/login/login.aspx? ReturnURL=https://www.nccn.org/professionals/physician_gls/pdf/pain.pdf. Accessed January 29, 2016.

45. US Food and Drug Administration. Risk evaluation and mitigation strategy (REMS) for extended-release and long-acting opioids. Available at: http://www. fda.gov/Drugs/DrugSafety/InformationbyDrugClass/ucm163647.htm. Accessed January 29, 2016.

46. Starrels JL, Becker WC, Alford DP, et al. Systematic review: treatment agreements and urine drug testing to reduce opioid misuse in patients with chronic pain. Ann Intern Med 2010;152(11):712–20.

47. Walsh AF, Broglio K. Pain management in advanced illness and comorbid substance use disorder. J Hosp Palliat Nurs 2010;12(1):8–14.

48. National Institute of Drug Abuse. Sample patient agreement forms. N.D. Available at: https://www.drugabuse.gov/sites/default/files/files/SamplePatientAgreementForms. pdf. Accessed February 6, 2016.

49. Owen GT, Burton AW, Schade CM, et al. Urine drug testing: current recommendations and best practices. Pain Physician 2012;15(3 Suppl):ES119-33.

50. Atluri S, Akbik H, Sudarshan G. Prevention of opioid abuse in chronic non-cancer pain: an algorithmic, evidence based approach. Pain Physician 2012;15(3 Suppl):ES177–89.

51. Prescription Drug Monitoring Program Center of Excellence at Brandeis. Status of prescription drug monitoring programs (PDMPS). 2014. Available at: http://www. pdmpassist.org/pdf/PDMPProgramStatus2014.pdf. Accessed January 29, 2016.

52. Reifler LM, Droz D, Bailey JE, et al. Do prescription monitoring programs impact state trends in opioid abuse/misuse? Pain Med 2012;13(3):434–42.

53. Prescription Drug Monitoring Program Center of Excellence at Brandeis. Mandating PDMP participation by medical providers: current status and experience in selected states. 2014. Available at: http://www.pdmpexcellence.org/ sites/all/pdfs/COE_briefing_mandates_2nd_rev.pdf. Accessed January 29, 2016.

54. New York State Department of Health Bureau of Narcotic Enforcement. Frequently asked questions for the NYS prescription monitoring program registry. 2014. Available at: http://www.health.ny.gov/professionals/narcotic/prescription_monitoring/docs/pmp_registry_faq.pdf. Accessed February 6, 2016.

55. McCluskey PD. Escrips seen as a way to combat opioid abuse. Boston Globe; 2015. Business. Available at: https://www.bostonglobe.com/business/2015/08/11/scripts-could-combat-opioid-overdose deluge/1PMGStb8tgdVc8eHDAde7N/story.html. Accessed June 3, 2016.

56. Lowes R. E-prescribing controlled substances now legal nationwide. Medscape Med News 2016.

57. New York State Department of Health. Frequently asked questions for electronic prescribing of controlled substances. 2016. Available at: https://www.health.ny.gov/professionals/narcotic/electronic_prescribing/docs/epcs_faqs.pdf. Accessed February 7, 2016.

58. Nicholson B. Primary care considerations of the pharmacokinetics and clinical use of extended-release opioids in treating patients with chronic noncancer pain. Postgrad Med 2013;125(1):115–27.

59. U.S. Department of Health and Human Services, FDA, CDER. Abuse-deterrent opioids—evaluation and labeling guidance for industry. 2015. Available at: http://www.fda.gov/downloads/drugs/guidancecomplianceregulatoryinformation/guidances/ucm334743.pdf. Accessed June 3, 2016.

60. Stanos S. Continuing evolution of opioid use in primary care practice: implications of emerging technologies. Curr Med Res Opin 2012;28(9):1505–16.

61. Substance Abuse and Mental Health Services Administration. SAMHSA opioid overdose prevention toolkit. Vol HHS Publication No. (SMA) 13–4742. Rockville (MD): Substance Abuse and Mental Health Services Administration; 2013.

62. Calas T, Wilkins M, Oliphant CM. Naloxone: an opportunity for another chance. J Nurs Pract 2016;12(3):154–60.

63. US Food and Drug Administration. Medication disposal: questions and answers. 2015. Available at: http://www.fda.gov/Drugs/ResourcesForYou/Consumers/BuyingUsingMedicineSafely/EnsuringSafeUseofMedicine/SafeDisposalofMedicines/ucm186188.htm. Accessed February 5, 2016.

64. US Department of Justice DEA, Office of Diversion Control. National take-back initiative. N.D. Available at: http://www.deadiversion.usdoj.gov/drug_disposal/takeback/index.html. Accessed February 6, 2016.

65. Wuhrman E, Broglio K. Patient-controlled analgesia helps manage pain. Nurs Crit Care 2015;10(4):38–42.

A Review of Palliative Sedation

Barton Bobb, MSN, FNP-BC, ACHPN

KEYWORDS

- Palliative sedation • End of life • Refractory symptoms • Midazolam
- Proportionate sedation

KEY POINTS

- Palliative sedation is a procedure used to treat refractory symptoms at end of life.
- Dyspnea and delirium are the most common physical symptoms addressed with palliative sedation, followed by pain and vomiting.
- The goal of palliative sedation is to alleviate intractable symptoms, but never to hasten the dying process, and it has not been found to do so.
- The process of palliative sedation continues to be surrounded by potential ethical concerns that are best discussed with patient and family before initiation.

INTRODUCTION

In spite of aggressive palliative measures, symptom management can sometimes become challenging at end of life. For these instances in which symptoms become refractory to standard treatment measures, the option of palliative sedation may be considered. The phrase terminal sedation was previously used, but was discontinued because the term implied that the goal was to shorten life.[1] The goal of palliative sedation is to relieve pain and suffering, never to shorten life. Systematic reviews of research involving the use of palliative sedation indicate that this intervention does not shorten patients' survival.[2,3] Two of the most common physical symptoms treated with palliative sedation are dyspnea and delirium.[2,4] Using palliative sedation to manage refractory nonphysical symptoms such as existential distress is less common and a more controversial practice that continues to be a topic of debate.[5–7]

CASE STUDY

M.B. is a 48-year-old man with advanced non–small cell lung carcinoma. He has been administered 3 lines of chemotherapy, multiple lung resections, and extensive

Disclosures: The author has no financial disclosures or conflicts of interest.
Thomas Palliative Care Services, Massey Cancer Center, Virginia Commonwealth University Health System, 1300 East Marshall Street, Richmond, VA 23298, USA
E-mail address: barton.bobb@vcuhealth.org

Nurs Clin N Am 51 (2016) 449–457
http://dx.doi.org/10.1016/j.cnur.2016.05.008
0029-6465/16/$ – see front matter © 2016 Elsevier Inc. All rights reserved.
nursing.theclinics.com

radiation therapy to treat his cancer aggressively as has continued to spread throughout his body, including bone and brain. However, at the end of his third line of chemotherapy, M.B. and his wife meet with his oncologist to discuss his goals. The decision is made to forego any further aggressive antineoplastic treatments because the cancer is continuing to grow and M.B. is experiencing worsening side effects from treatment and a decline in his functional status.

He enrolls in home hospice after having a drainage catheter system placed to drain recurrent pleural fluid collections. His appetite gradually increases as his nausea decreases after stopping chemotherapy. His home hospice nurses continue to help with draining the pleural fluid and adjusting his opioids/other medications that control his chronic cancer-related pain and shortness of breath. As he continues to decline over time, he ultimately becomes bed bound and less and less responsive. He complains of worsening shortness of breath and shows signs of hyperactive delirium.

When escalating doses of sublingual injectable haloperidol, followed by injectable lorazepam, both scheduled and as needed, fail to control his delirium and worsening work of breathing, M.B. is admitted to an inpatient palliative care unit at a local hospital. With informed consent from his wife, continuous palliative sedation is initiated with a continuous midazolam infusion and boluses as needed administered by the nursing staff. The continuous rate is adjusted every 4 hours as needed based on how many boluses he requires in a 4-hour period. After approximately 8 hours of titration, M.B. at last seems to be comfortable, with unlabored breathing and only occasional, slight signs of the previously uncontrolled hyperactive delirium. A day later, M.B. dies peacefully with his wife and children at his bedside.

TERMINOLOGY, INDICATIONS, AND TYPES OF PALLIATIVE SEDATION
Evolving Definitions

As mentioned earlier, the term palliative sedation has evolved over time. The first reference to this procedure at end of life was terminal sedation, to differentiate it from other forms of sedation.[8] In a review of research findings, palliative sedation was found to alleviate pain and suffering, and not to hasten death,[2,3] and so this definition was deemed to be misleading and incorrect.[1] Although some other phrases for sedation at end of life, such as total sedation, sedation for intractable symptoms, and controversially even slow euthanasia, are also used at times, palliative sedation is the term most commonly used at present in most research studies.[1,8]

Indications for the Use of Palliative Sedation

Palliative sedation is used when terminally ill patients experience uncontrolled symptoms refractory to escalating standard treatment regimens at the end of life. At what point a symptom is considered refractory is not always clear and is discussed later, but a frequently used, general description is a symptom "for which all possible treatment has failed, or it is estimated that no methods are available for palliation within the time frame and risk: benefit ratio that the patient can tolerate."[1] Another definition of palliative sedation entails treating symptoms "that cannot be adequately controlled in a tolerable time frame despite aggressive use of usual therapies and that seems unlikely to be adequately controlled by further invasive or noninvasive therapies without excessive or intolerable acute or chronic side effects."[8(p441)]

The timing for the initiation of palliative sedation has not been clearly determined. In general, expert clinicians agree that patients with refractory symptoms with prognoses of hours to days are considered most appropriate for continuous sedation, although intermittent sedation may be used earlier.[5]

Palliative sedation is most commonly used to manage refractory physical symptoms for terminally ill patients with cancer, dyspnea and delirium in particular, but nonphysical symptoms and existential suffering can potentially be treated in specific circumstances.[2–4] Pain and vomiting are two of the additional common physical symptoms at end of life that may require palliative sedation.[2,8] In a 2012 systematic literature review of palliative sedation used in terminally ill patients with cancer over a 30-year span, 54% of the 774 sedated patients received palliative sedation for delirium, 30% for dyspnea, 17% for pain, and 5% for vomiting.[2] In the same review, 19% of patients received palliative sedation for nonphysical symptoms, broadly categorized as psychological distress.[2] However, using palliative sedation for nonphysical symptoms (eg, anxiety, hopelessness, fear) or existential suffering remains a controversial topic, and is also be discussed further later.[8] **Box 1** lists common symptoms managed with palliative sedation.

Types of Sedation to Achieve Palliative Sedation

Palliative sedation can be achieved by several methods. To decide on which method is most likely to be effective, practitioners may need to consider several factors, such as the nature, onset, and severity of the patient's symptoms, the patient's overall prognosis, and the goals and wishes of the patient/family.[1]

With regard to the extent of sedation necessary, the principle of proportionality mandates that the patient's consciousness be reduced to the level necessary to relieve the refractory suffering adequately. This principle helps guide the initiation and titration of palliative sedation.[1,8,9] The goal is to preserve the patient's ability to interact with loved ones as much as possible while obtaining adequate symptom control and comfort with the lowest level of sedation necessary. The type of sedation used may therefore range from only light/superficial sedation to deep sedation and is administered either intermittently or continuously.[1,10] Such sedation should be achieved with the use of a sedative or anesthetic, with the aim of sedation, not by simply increasing medications previously used to control symptoms (eg, opioids) until the sedating side effect causes oversedation. This latter technique can lead to unwanted side effects (eg, myoclonus, nausea).[1,10]

For sudden and severe symptoms at end of life, such as massive bleeding, terminal air hunger, or excruciating pain crisis, sudden/emergency sedation may need to be used.[10,11] In this situation, aggressive, deep, and continuous sedation may need to be used rapidly to alleviate suffering in an imminently dying patient. A contingency treatment plan, both in the inpatient and outpatient setting, should be in place in the event of a catastrophic event, such as might occur if head and neck cancer extends into the external carotid artery. Temporary respite sedation may also achieve the rapid relief necessary for terminally ill patients with uncontrolled symptoms that may later

---

Box 1
Refractory symptoms commonly managed with palliative sedation

- Delirium
- Dyspnea
- Pain
- Vomiting
- Nonphysical symptoms (psychological distress and existential suffering)

Data from Refs.[2–4,8]

respond to potential additional treatments.[11] Patients are monitored closely while sedated with the goal of restoring them to their prior level of consciousness in order to resume trying to find other treatment options.[11]

TREATMENT OPTIONS
Pharmacologic and Nonpharmacologic

Benzodiazepines, especially midazolam, remain the mainstay of treatment of palliative sedation.[1,2,5,11] Midazolam is widely used because it has a fast onset but also a short half-life, which allows rapid titration and may be given intravenously or subcutaneously.[1,5,11] Midazolam has sedative/hypnotic, anxiolytic, antispasmodic/muscle relaxant, and anticonvulsant properties.[1,2,5] It can be given together with opioids or haloperidol, plus it can also be reversed with flumazenil if needed.[11] Lorazepam is a longer-acting benzodiazepine than midazolam that can also be given orally or sublingually in liquid form.[8] Its elimination is not affected by hepatic or renal insufficiency.[5] It is therefore a better choice for use in home hospice and is often part of the hospice symptom management kit, potentially in concentrated formulation.

Other medications commonly used for palliative sedation include the antipsychotic chlorpromazine, barbiturates (phenobarbital or pentobarbital primarily), and the anesthetic propofol.[1,8,11] Although the antipsychotic haloperidol has been used for palliative sedation, it is usually not sedating enough to be an effective option for palliative sedation.[1] **Box 2** lists medications commonly used for palliative sedation.

When palliative sedation is administered, any other medications previously given for symptom management can, and usually should, be continued (eg, opioids for dyspnea, haloperidol for delirium), but they are usually no longer uptitrated once palliative sedation is initiated in order to avoid potential side effects.

Although there are no specific nonpharmacologic treatments to help with palliative sedation, besides providing excellent nursing care, any nonpharmacologic treatments previously used for the refractory symptom being treated with palliative sedation should be continued. For example, the use of a fan blowing across the face has been found to have a positive effect for the treatment of dyspnea.[12]

Treatment Guidelines and Position Statements

Many national and international organizations, such as the American Medical Association, European Association for Palliative Care, National Hospice and Palliative Care

---

Box 2
Summary of most commonly used drugs for palliative sedation and basic starting dosage range

- Midazolam, 0.5 to 1 mg/h intravenous (IV)/subcutaneous (SC) starting infusion dose, 0.5 to 5 mg as needed or loading dose

- Lorazepam, 0.5 to 5 mg oral/IV/sublingual dose every 1 to 2 hours as needed, every 4 to 6 hours scheduled

- Chlorpromazine, 12.5 to 25 mg IV/IM dose every 2 to 4 hours, 25 to 100 mg per rectum every 4 to 12 hours

- Phenobarbital, 1 to 3 mg/kg IV/SC loading dose followed by 0.5 mg/kg/h infusion

- Propofol, 20 mg IV loading dose followed by continuous infusion of 10 mg/h or 2.5 to 5 μg/kg/min and increase by 10 to 20 mg/h every 10 minutes as needed

Data from Refs.[1,8,11]

Organization, and the European Society for Medical Oncology, have published guidelines or position papers on palliative sedation.[5,11] Several systematic literature reviews have been published comparing these guidelines and have concluded that wide variance exists in most aspects of palliative sedation.[5,13,14]

Several nursing organizations, including Hospice and Palliative Nurses Association (HPNA), American Nurses Association (ANA), and American Society for Pain Management Nursing (ASPMN), have position statements about nursing care at end of life.[5,15,16] The HPNA statement specifically focuses on palliative sedation for patients with intractable suffering, including physical and nonphysical/existential symptoms, who are imminently dying (hours to days left to live).[5] The ANA and ASPMN statements do not specifically address the practice of palliative sedation, but they both advocate for patients' right to relief of pain and other symptoms, without artificial life-prolonging measures in accordance with patients' wishes, at end of life.[15,16]

ETHICAL CONSIDERATIONS

Although the procedure of palliative sedation has become widely accepted and practiced throughout the United States and other parts of the world, there continues to exist a range of ethical questions surrounding certain aspects of the practice of palliative sedation.

Proportionality, Euthanasia, and the Principle of Double Effect

As previously discussed, palliative sedation is usually started with a proportionate approach that uses the least amount of sedation necessary to relieve intractable suffering and is only initiated after careful deliberation of the goals of care.[1,9,11,17] The goal is never to hasten a patient's death, which stands in contrast with both euthanasia and physician-assisted suicide.[11,17] In some cases, artificial nutrition and hydration (ANH) may also be continued in the interim until palliative sedation can potentially be discontinued or it becomes more evident that death is becoming imminent. Potential risks versus benefits should always be weighed carefully when deciding whether to continue or stop ANH.[11,17]

When deep continuous sedation is used to treat multiple refractory symptoms at end of life, and no ANH is provided, the goal is not to hasten death, and available evidence on the use of palliative sedation indicates that death is not hastened.[2,3] Therefore, apparently it is not necessary to invoke the ethical principle of double effect (the principle that states that hastening death is justified when it is an inadvertent side effect of treating refractory symptoms at end of life).[1] Nevertheless, the initiation of aggressive, deep, continuous palliative sedation is never done lightly and is a last resort to alleviate extreme, refractory suffering in dying patients. The medical ethical principle of beneficence, to do good, while also ensuring nonmaleficence (not doing harm), should always be fulfilled.[11]

When is a Symptom Considered to be Refractory?

Even though there are previously mentioned definitions of what constitutes a refractory symptom, there are no clearly delineated criteria that allow providers to make a definitive determination of when a symptom has been treated extensively enough to be considered refractory. In some instances, palliative sedation could be used prematurely or for an inappropriate indication; examples include overlooking a potentially reversible cause, using palliative sedation out of exhaustion and frustration over caring for a challenging symptomatic patient, or failing to consult experts who could potentially help relieve the refractory symptoms.[11] An example is omitting to involve interdisciplinary team members to help assess and treat a patient with severe psychological or existential distress before resorting to palliative sedation; this is a situation in which the use of palliative sedation remains highly controversial.

Informed Consent Before Initiation

It is standard practice to obtain informed consent and document it in the patient's medical record before starting palliative sedation. Patient autonomy is to be respected whenever possible, as is the use of substitutionary decision making by legal next of kin/designated surrogate decision makers if the patient cannot participate in the discussion or chooses not to.[1,8,11] Ideally, informed consent should be obtained from the patient before it becomes necessary to initiate palliative sedation, preferably with any family/surrogate decision maker in attendance with the patient's permission.[8,11] The patient's wishes can then be honored most accurately, even if the patient is no longer able to clearly speak when palliative sedation is indicated.

Key pieces of information during the informed consent process, which should be provided in a calm and compassionate manner during a family meeting, include the patient's current condition, prognosis, nature of the refractory symptoms and why it is thought that there are no further conventional treatment options available to obtain adequate symptom control, risks versus benefits of palliative sedation, and details about the palliative sedation process with predetermined goals of sedation.[8,11]

Nonphysiologic Symptoms/Existential Distress: to Use or Not to Use Palliative Sedation?

One of the most controversial questions regarding palliative sedation is whether to use this procedure to potentially control nonphysiologic symptoms such as existential distress. Existential distress may be characterized by "feelings of helplessness, hopelessness, and fear of death."[5(p666)] Because existential suffering is not universally defined or clearly understood, it is difficult for health care professionals to assess its intractable nature, let alone provide adequate treatment of it.[18] Extreme caution should therefore be exercised before seriously considering palliative sedation, especially continuous, deep sedation, as a viable treatment of existential suffering.[7] Should the possibility of palliative sedation be requested/considered for a patient with refractory existential suffering, it is important to review current professional position statements, have an institutional policy in place, and to seek the guidance of an ethics committee before giving this proposal serious consideration.

NURSING CARE
Before Initiating Palliative Sedation

The patient's nurse, whether at home or in a hospital, plays an important role during the process of initiating palliative sedation. Nurses are often in a unique position to establish close rapport with patients and their families. Because nurses are usually the health care providers who spend the most time at the patient's bedside, they often develop a deep level of trust with and knowledge about patients and their families, including their goals and wishes, which serve to guide the plan of care, particularly with regard to palliative care. Nurses may also have the most insight into the extent of the patients' suffering and lack of response to treatments, which serves as the entry point for discussions related to the potential need for palliative sedation.

If the decision is made to formally pursue palliative sedation, the nurse is ideally present during the patient/family meeting as the primary provider obtains informed consent. The nurse's presence lends additional support to the patient/family and also serves as a bridge to help foster additional trust in, and partnership with, the primary provider. If there are additional questions after the meeting, which there most likely will be, the nurse is aware of what was discussed in the meeting and can help clarify any questions or pass them on to the provider. The nurse can also provide calming, nonjudgmental reassurance and encouragement to the patient/family that they are making the correct decision, and that the nurse will work hard to help achieve the desired comfort for the patient and will also continue to answer questions about how the process of palliative sedation will proceed. If the process of palliative sedation is discussed and started in a more urgent manner, it is of utmost importance that the nurse maintains a calm and reassuring demeanor so that the patient and family feel supported in this difficult time.

During the Process of Palliative Sedation

First and foremost, the nurse taking care of the patient receiving palliative sedation must be vigilant and attentive to monitoring the patient's level of comfort and giving additional medication as needed. There should be clear expectations of what the goals of palliative sedation are and how the nurse can assess for the patient's adequate level of comfort, unless the patient is still able to self-report the degree of symptom control. If the treatments being given are not providing the desired effect, or are not well tolerated, the patient should be proactive in approaching the primary team about changing orders as needed. The patient will be able to provide detailed data from the bedside, and also will often have suggestions on potential adjustments/changes ready, to be able to provide guidance to the primary team about the next potential course of action, to include only slight medication adjustments. In contrast, the nurse may be monitoring for improvement in symptoms to the extent that it may become possible to start weaning the patient off the anesthetic or sedative, if that is an established goal for this particular patient.

The nurse also gives attention to the patient's comfort in a variety of other ways, especially for patients who are no longer able to make their needs known. Some of the nursing care components would then resemble those of other comatose/semicomatose patients at end of life. The nurse monitors for bowel and bladder function and places a urinary catheter if indicated. Continued regular turning/repositioning for comfort and good oral care (eg, with mouth swabs) are also important, and are things that family members at the bedside can also be instructed in performing, and may give them a sense of purpose and control in this difficult time. In the home setting, they are usually the primary bedside caregivers so it is imperative that they feel empowered and comfortable performing all hands-on care. The nurse can also encourage family members to continue interacting and communicating with their loved one, as would be done with any patient in the last hours of life.

The nurse can also assess for ways to make the patient's environment more homelike and comforting for the patient, especially in a hospital setting. For example, the nurse can ask the family to bring in some of the patient's favorite music to play, pictures to put up at the bedside, or a special blanket to use from home. Ancillary/complementary services, such as music therapy, pet therapy, aromatherapy, chaplain, and other volunteer services, may also add some comfort for both the patient and family. Some volunteers are also trained in memory making/living legacy work to help patients/families cope with the impending death and make meaning of it. The nurse can also ensure that the ambient temperature and lighting are appropriate and use some of the other previously mentioned nonpharmacologic measures to help with symptom control.

Throughout this process, bedside nurses can be instrumental in assessing patients and their families for any questions they may have or any unmet needs that they may not verbalize. The nurse may need to explain what signs and symptoms signify impending death and validate any concerns as death draws near. The family may even question their treatment decisions and require more information and reassurance. If nurses are unable to answer certain questions, they can pass along any other concerns or observations. Nurses should continue to support families throughout this time, especially if their loved one is actively dying. As with other patients who are actively dying, nurses can encourage the family to participate in the hands-on care of their loved one (eg, repositioning, oral care, grooming, or massage). They may also help foster reminiscing or engaging in other forms of memory making. Patients may have dreams/visions that can be discussed.

After Palliative Sedation

If palliative sedation has been stopped because the patient is feeling better and no longer requires it, the bedside nurse should reassure the patient and family that the nurse will assess and treat any signs of recurrence. If the patient has died, the nurse will spend a significant amount of time with routine postmortem care, which includes notifying the covering physician to pronounce the patient, calling the LifeNet organ donation organization, paging the chaplain, notifying decedent affairs, and preparing the body for transportation to the morgue. Family may choose to be involved in postmortem care, with the assistance of the nurse as needed. The nurse is instrumental in providing support and comfort to the loved ones who are grieving their loss. It is likely to be especially important to remind the family that they made the right decision in asking for palliative sedation at their loved one's end of life and that it was necessary to ensure their comfort without hastening their dying.

Last but not least, the nurses caring for the patient receiving palliative sedation, especially those who spent the most time with the patient and the nurse responsible at the patient's death, should make sure they are able to debrief about the process and find ways to allow themselves some extra self-care. The unit chaplain may be called on to check on staff more frequently and specifically ask about how they are feeling about their experience caring for the patient receiving palliative sedation. Occasionally, the chaplain may be needed to lead a debriefing session. Nurses were found to have higher level of comfort in their roles during the process of palliative sedation when they knew more about the personal life of the patient and took pride in the interdisciplinary team process.[8]

SUMMARY

Palliative sedation has become an established palliative procedure designed to alleviate refractory pain and suffering, primarily from physical symptoms such as dyspnea and delirium, at the end of life. This procedure is not intended to, and does not, hasten the dying process. Benzodiazepines are the most frequently used drugs to initiate palliative sedation. Ethical concerns about the proper use of this procedure, especially when used for existential suffering, continue to be debated extensively. Nurses play a vital role in helping ensure that this procedure goes smoothly and that both patients and families are comfortable throughout this difficult process.

REFERENCES

1. Maltoni M, Setola E. Palliative sedation in patients with cancer. Cancer Control 2015;22(4):433–44.
2. Maltoni M, Scarpi E, Rosat M, et al. Palliative sedation in end-of-life care and survival: a systematic review. J Clin Oncol 2012;30(12):1378–83.

3. Beller E, van Driel M, McGregor L, et al. Palliative pharmacological sedation for terminally ill adults. Cochrane Database Syst Rev 2015;(1):CD010206.
4. Claessens P, Menten J, Schotsmans P, et al. Palliative sedation: a review of the recent literature. J Pain Symptom Manage 2008;36(3):310–33.
5. Gurschick L, Mayer D, Hanson L. Palliative sedation: an analysis of international guidelines and position statements. Am J Hosp Palliat Care 2015;32(6):660–71.
6. Swart S, van der Heide A, Zuylen L, et al. Continuous palliative sedation: not only a response to physical suffering. J Palliat Med 2014;17(1):27–36.
7. Bruce A, Boston P. Relieving existential suffering through palliative sedation: discussion of an uneasy practice. J Adv Nurs 2011;67(12):2732–40.
8. Knight P, Espinosa L, Freeman B. Sedation for refractory symptoms. In: Ferrell B, Coyle N, Pace J, editors. Oxford textbook of palliative nursing. Oxford (United Kingdom), New York: Oxford University Press; 2015. p. 440–8.
9. Berger J. The proportionate value of proportionality in palliative sedation. J Clin Ethics 2014;25(3):219–21.
10. Lossignol D. End-of-life sedation: is there an alternative? Curr Opin Oncol 2015; 27(4):358–64.
11. Cherny N. ESMO clinical practice guidelines for the management of refractory symptoms at the end of life and the use of palliative sedation. Ann Oncol 2014; 25(Suppl 3):iii143–52.
12. Galbraith S, Fagan P, Perkins P, et al. Does the use of a handheld fan improve chronic dyspnea? A randomized, controlled, crossover trial. J Pain Symptom Manage 2010;39(5):831–8.
13. Schildmann E, Schildmann J. Palliative sedation therapy: a systematic literature review and critical appraisal of available guidance on indication and decision making. J Palliat Med 2014;17(5):601–11.
14. Schildmann E, Schildmann J, Kiesewetter I. Medication and monitoring in palliative sedation therapy: a systematic review and quality assessment of published guidelines. J Pain Symptom Manage 2015;49(4):734–46.
15. Reynolds J, Drew D, Dunoody C. American Society for Pain Management Nursing position statement: pain management at the end of life. Pain Manag Nurs 2013; 14(3):172–5.
16. American Nurses Association (ANA). Registered nurses' roles and responsibilities in providing expert care and counseling at the end of life. 2010. Available at: http://www.nursingworld.org/MainMenuCategories/ EthicsStandards/Ethics-Position-Statements/etpain14426.pdf. Accessed April 24, 2016.
17. Kirk T, Mahon M. National Hospice and Palliative Care Organization (NHPOCO) position statement and commentary on the use of palliative sedation in imminently dying terminally ill patients. J Pain Symptom Manage 2010;39(5):914–23.
18. Sadler K. Palliative sedation to alleviate existential suffering at end-of-life: Insight into a controversial practice. Can Oncol Nurs J 2012;22(3):195–9.

Family Care During End-of-Life Vigils

Colleen Fleming-Damon, PhDc, APRN-BC, ACHPN, CT[a,b],*

KEYWORDS

- Vigil • End of life • Family • Nursing care

KEY POINTS

- The family vigil at the end of life is a complex human experience.
- Nurses are often present and bear witness to family vigils at end of life.
- The vigil experience has the potential for human suffering or the potential for growth.
- Nursing care during the vigil experience may lead to positive outcomes for family.

INTRODUCTION

An end-of-life vigil is the act of being with another toward death. A family vigil at end of life is a phenomenon that occurs when significant others gather by the bedside of dying individuals in the weeks, days, or hours prior to the death event. It is not unusual for nurses who minister to the dying to be present, bear witness, and share in this human experience. The purpose of this article is to review seminal and current research regarding the meaning and structure of the lived experience of vigil keeping for a dying family member, and to translate this research to inform nursing practice regarding family care during the transition at end of life.

BACKGROUND

Dying and death are universally lived experiences. In the United States, approximately 2.4 million Americans die each year, including an estimated 43% who will die in a hospital, 22% who will die in a skilled nursing facility, 25% who will die at home, and 10% who will die in other settings.[1] These individuals may have family or significant others who keep vigil during the transition of dying and death, exhibiting diverse interactional and emotional responses to the dying–death experience. These may include closed awareness, separation anxiety, spiritual distress, existential aloneness, and negative

Disclosure: None.
[a] MJHS Institute for Innovation in Palliative Care, 39 Broadway, New York, NY 10006, USA;
[b] Adelphi University, 1 South Avenue, Garden City, NY 11530, USA
* 121 Brimstone Hill Road, Pine Bush, NY 12566.
E-mail address: fleming-damon@adelphi.edu

emotions such as bewilderment, denial, anger, sadness, disappointment, resentment, guilt, exhaustion, and desperation.[1–10]

In contrast to these negative responses, some studies report positive responses to approaching death that are experienced by patients and families, such as open awareness, spirituality, family support, autonomy, hope, meaningful purpose in life, and peaceful acceptance.[11–13] The experience of vigil keeping while approaching loss is described as a complex phenomenon for individuals and families at the end of life, and for the nurses who provide care for them.

SIGNIFICANCE TO NURSING

End-of-life care is an important focus and essential to nursing practice.[9,14,15] The end-of-life experience has the potential for human suffering, or the potential for growth.[13,16,17] These diverse outcomes emphasize the importance of providing quality nursing care to dying individuals and their families during the vigil experience. Yet, many nurses lack the necessary education and preparation to provide this specialized care.[10,18,19] Integrating palliative care into nursing education will better prepare nurses in their multiple roles as caregiver, advocate, and guide, and enhance care to patients and families during the vigil experience.[9,10,19,20]

Keeping vigil at the end-of-life is a powerful transitional process experienced by families. It presents families with a time of crisis, while concurrently presenting potential opportunity for growth and positive change. It is a transition that can lead families to outcomes of stagnation and continued suffering, or movement toward the possibility of healing and transformation.[13,21] Often, nurses share in this experience, and are present at the bedside, vigiling with families of dying individuals. Nursing education on end-of-life care, coupled with an informed presence at the bedside, can enable nurses the opportunity to guide and facilitate this family transition with positive outcomes. It is the nursing profession's historical, theoretical, and philosophical underpinnings that support a holistic model of caring science and define nurses as compassionate caregivers across the continuum of wellness, illness, dying, and death.

LITERATURE REVIEW

A search and review of the research literature were conducted to identify primary research studies on the phenomenon of family vigil keeping. The databases of EBSCOhost, Ovid Medline, and Psych Info were searched between the periods of 1995 to 2016, for research studies published in peer-reviewed journals from various disciplines, using the specific keyword "vigil." There were 66 papers found with the specific term of "vigil." Narrowing with advanced search methods using the specific keywords "vigil keeping, family," and "death and dying," 5 research studies on family vigil keeping were identified. The following is a review of these 5 studies, the conceptual definitions, and a synthesis of the literature on the phenomenon of family vigil keeping at the end of life.

CONCEPTUAL DEFINITIONS

The concept of "family" is defined as 1 or more close others, either blood- or non-blood- related, defined as family by the dying individual. The term "end of life" is defined as a state when an individual's recovery from an illness cannot be expected, and death is considered to be inevitable and imminent. The selection of the term "vigiling" indicates ongoing action in the ever-changing, dynamic process of the vigil experience, in contrast to a static or episodic event.

VIGIL AS TRANSITION

In 1 phenomenological study on meaning of the transition experience from medical care to palliative care for 100 advanced cancer patients in 6 European cities, Larkin, De Casterle, and Schotsman discovered emergent themes reflective of the meaning and impact of transition.[22] The first theme was "lived body" instability, and the human response of seeking restoration. The second theme was the "lived space" of impermanence and the human response of seeking or creating a secure space. The third theme was "lived time," or oscillation in the liminal space between the present life situation and the uncertainty of the future, and the human response of negotiating time. The fourth theme was the "lived other," with shifting relational bonds and the human response of forming, renewing, rebalancing, and relinquishing relationships at the end of life. The final overarching theme was "living transiently in the shadow of death."[22]

Davies conducted a qualitative study with 71 family members to explore the lived experience of a family unit with advanced cancer in 1 member. The essential thematic description that resulted was: "the transition of fading away."[8] Transition is described as a universal concept reflecting the human lived experience when change occurs. The transition of fading away is comprised of 7 interrelated and intertwined components: redefining, burdening, struggling with paradox, contending with change, searching for meaning, living day to day, and preparing for death. Dying and death represent inevitable change within the individual and family system. The end-of-life vigil presents such a transition for families.

VIGIL: A STATE OF AWARENESS

In a landmark study regarding the process of dying in 6 San Francisco hospitals, Glaser and Strauss discovered contexts of death awareness in individuals, families, and caregivers at end of life.[3] The researchers defined awareness of dying as a mutual knowledge and recognition of an individual's defined status of dying, and the context within which these people interact while taking cognizance of their status. The contexts of awareness identified are categorized as closed awareness, suspected awareness, mutual pretense, awareness, and open awareness. The researchers proposed that with open awareness, individuals and their family members are empowered to plan an end-of-life vigil setting, including people present and the rites and rituals of family preference.

Glaser and Strauss provide a view on family transition from a state of unawareness to a state of awareness of death, which may be prompted by disclosure of hospital staff, or observed cognitive or physical changes that are obvious to the family. The study participants reported that awareness of death provided the impetus for change in family behaviors, including

Notification of extended family
Increased visiting time with attendance by family members and significant others
Increased attention patterns toward the individual dying
Increased family need for information
Focused family decision-making regarding treatment versus comfort measures
Negotiation and management of private space
Family preparation for death

In summary, individual and family awareness provide the impetus for assembling and keeping vigil for a dying family member.

VIGIL AS PSYCHOLOGICAL CONSTRUCT

Kastenbaum describes the deathbed scene during the final hours or days of life as a psychosocial transition that is constructed mentally through the use of a family narrative.[23,24] Narratives may provide ways of preserving mental constructs of direct encounters with mortality. Through hermeneutic review of multiple hospice case histories, the researcher constructed the unfolding of a deathbed scene. The onset of the deathbed scene begins with the signs or signals of physical decline and resultant family perception that either the individual is dying or experiencing a medical crisis that may be reversed. Each of these perceptions is a formulated construct. Some families may be united or divided regarding these alternative cognitive constructions. Both constructs provide the impetus for vigilance, a shared culture that provides symbols and meaning modules that include keeping watch or being on guard during a crisis.

Kastenbaum's case study analysis asserts that over several months after the death event, family members may select, choose, and refine their narratives, with most families arriving at a fairly stable and consistent construction and meaning of the deathbed experience. It becomes the story of a family event, the totality of the group experience. The researcher describes that the family narrative will unfold in the framework of transition in that there will be a beginning, an interval of evolutional psychosocial development, a movement to a state of conflict or chaos, and resolution or denouement toward a meaningful symbolic structure and meaning.

VIGIL AS A PSYCHOLOGICAL PROCESS

Qualitative research conducted with a direct focus on the phenomenon of vigil keeping describes vigil as a psychological process.[25] Kuisle explored the meaning and experience of vigil keeping with 11 individuals, and results describe vigil as an internal place where one may wait and watch for whatever comes. In terms of emergent themes, the researcher describes a transition of moving into a state of vigil, with waiting, alertness, silence, and holding the tension of opposites from darkness to light, from night to day, in uncertainty with the possibility of transformation. This vigil study is a significant contribution to research in that vigil is examined directly and presented from an individual, internal, and conscious–unconscious psychological perspective. Nursing research supports the assertion that vigil keeping is a psychological process for family members.

Phillips and Reed also conducted a qualitative study to understand family caregivers' perspectives of providing end-of-life care to elders facing expected deaths from life-limiting, chronic illnesses. The study design incorporated grounded theory with in-depth interviews with 27 participants, 13 spouses, and 14 children. Eight core characteristics or themes of end-of-life caregiving were extracted from the data. End-of-life caregiving was found to be: unpredictable, intense, complex, frightening, anguishing, profoundly moving, affirming, and dissolving familiar social boundaries. These core characteristics unified into an essential theme expressed in the words of one caregiver as "jumping into the abyss of someone else's dying," which reflects an underlying psychological process to the vigil experience.[26]

VIGIL AS ANTICIPATORY MOURNING

A vigil is time spent prior to a death event. Some studies found document a wide range of family responses in anticipation of a death. Anticipatory mourning has been defined as a process that includes deep or intense feelings of sorrow or distress, before a loss that may cause suffering.[6] Lindemann first identified the phenomenon of anticipatory grief as a syndrome of grief reactions in 101 individuals experiencing separation and threat of death.[27] Therefore, forewarning of death is a necessary condition to precede grief reaction, not an actual loss. Since the introduction of this concept, anticipatory mourning has been closely associated with transition from illness to dying and death.[28]

VIGIL: THE ACT OF VIGILANCE

Vigil has been defined as "the act or state of being constantly attentive or keeping careful in response to signs of opportunity, activity, or danger."[29] Vigil is the root word and origin of meaning for vigilance. If vigilance is the state, then vigil keeping may be perceived as the act of vigilance. In the research literature, vigilance has been conceptualized in diverse ways. Three thematic conceptual definitions can be derived from the phenomenon of vigilance described in nursing literature as: an expression of family caring through watchful awareness[30–32]; an interactive, social process with caring watchfulness, as evidenced by intensified connections and relationships[33,34]; and a complex multidimensional process of caring, through watching and observing for signs and managing illness with the purpose of protection and preservation of a family member's health and safety.[33–35]

VIGIL AS CARING

With the purpose of understanding family experiences of caring when a family member dies, Fridh, Forberg, and Bergbom conducted a study guided by phenomenological hermeneutic method.[36] Interviews with 17 family members of patients who had died in an intensive care unit were analyzed, with several emergent themes such as: "being confronted with the threat of loss, maintaining a vigil, trusting the care, adapting and trying to understand, facing death, the need for privacy and togetherness, and experiencing reconciliation."[36] This study is 1 of 3 nursing studies that identify vigil as an emergent theme. For the purpose of this focused article, the theme, "maintaining a vigil," is explored regarding family vigil.

According to families, a vigil commenced when there was an understanding that death was inevitable. They identified the need to be close and were protective of personal time with their dying family member. Many described with certainty that although sedated or unconscious, they perceived their family member could feel their presence. Families described feelings of tension and worry, which dissipated when focus shifted from their own emotions to the comfort of the individual dying. When the central focus was on their dying family member, all other matters seemed to be unimportant. Vigil behaviors included sitting long hours by the bedside in a state of watchful attention, while maintaining physical contact and verbal communication with the dying.[36]

The families described maintaining vigil as a private family experience. Members of the family had a need for proximity to their dying family member, information regarding the dying process, and for togetherness during the vigil that continued after death. Importantly, nurses were perceived as guides, piloting family through the vigil experience. According to families, piloting led to feelings of care, support, and comfort. A lack of piloting, as evidenced by a lack of caring relationships, the inability for close proximity to their loved one, or being excluded from information, led to feelings of loneliness and abandonment. The authors concluded that vigils that involved a caring relationship between nurse and family had a greater potential for higher satisfaction with care and better outcomes for the family in terms of coping and bereavement.[36]

VIGIL AS SOCIAL PROCESS

Read and Wuest conducted a study of 12 daughters caring for their dying elderly parents who died at home. What emerged was a substantive theory of relinquishing at end of life, including the subprocesses of keeping vigil, navigating systems, facing loss, and the end process of coming to terms. With a focus on processes of keeping vigil, family caregivers provide a close protective watchfulness of loved ones by monitoring patterns of illness and emergent needs. Vigils were described as "anticipated surveillance" for signals of threat to the dying individual and to family integrity. Vigils offer protection against these threats, thereby restoring a sense of control to the caregiver, and order in the context of perceived disorder.[37]

Williams and colleagues conducted a phenomenological study to explore the experience of being present at the hospital death of a family member in a Veterans Affairs Medical Center. Interviews were conducted with 78 recently bereaved wives and daughters of veterans who died in 6 medical centers in the southeast United States. Study results described *two* major themes from family member interviews that involved phases. The first phase is the phenomenon of "settling in," and the second phase is the phenomenon of "gathering around."[38]

Family participants describe settling in as the initial phase of hospitalization. Settling in involves family spending greater amounts of time visiting during the transition of dying and death. This time is spent maintaining a protective and nurturing presence in the hospital room of their dying family member. Sustaining an ongoing presence gives rise to everyday issues of physical, emotional, and spiritual sustenance for families, many of whom transform the hospital room into a home-like environment, bringing in possessions, engaging in familiar activities, and eliciting support from staff, who become honorary extended family members.

The second phase of gathering around describes the assembly of a wider circle of immediate and extended family members to the bedside as the patient nears death. At this juncture, the study mentions the concept of holding vigil. Vigil is described by the researchers as immediate family members remaining close by the patient, holding vigil around the clock, with extended family members and friends making visits of short duration to offer support or say goodbye. The study findings reveal that family vigils occur in greater frequency in the acute-care hospital setting. It is a time of uncertainty, and because the time frame of watching and waiting has no predetermined end, vigils can be an anxious, unsettling, and draining experience for family members.[38]

The family members described ways of being during vigils, as evidenced by family gathering and presence at the bedside of their loved one. The researchers noted ways of doing during vigils by the family actions such as waiting for death, watching for physical changes, performing rituals of prayer and song, and sharing of loving sentiments and tender goodbyes. The major theme and title of the study was what 1 family participant described as "a room full of chairs around the bed." The descriptor "around the bed" provides the image of a circle, without beginning or end. A circle may be symbolic of family connectedness, commitment, and unity.[38]

VIGIL AS RITUAL

Research describes the phenomenon of vigil as a human rite or ritual. A ritual has been defined as a sequence of activities involving gestures, words, and objects performed in a sequestered place and sequence of time.[39] These activities have been found to be symbolic and meaningful to lived human experience. Collective values, beliefs, and traditions create rituals as cultural constructs found within a human society. Rituals have been well documented within religious rites and ceremonies, and within rites of human passage or life transitions.[39] Vigils are described in various life transitions and are an observed phenomenon during the transition of dying and death. Rituals are created for the psychological wellbeing of individuals and for social order, for group unity in a dynamic cyclical pattern of chaos and order, and for the purpose of constructing meaning in human experience.[39–41]

SUMMATION OF RESEARCH

The search for meaning, structure, and form of family vigils in the interdisciplinary research literature offers support for the phenomenon. As a starting point of identifying the phenomenon, the research data present several descriptions:

A family vigil is a transition that begins with cognitive awareness of perceived or actual threat of death, with a conscious–unconscious psychosocial construct, increased vigilance, and initiation of social process.

Vigil is an act of vigilance, an act of caring, and an act of ritual. It is a time of anticipation, a time of diverse emotional responses inclusive to anticipatory mourning.

Vigiling presents as a complex phenomenon that has emerged as various themes in a few nursing studies. As a result, further nursing research with direct focus on end-of-life family vigil is clearly indicated.

NURSING IMPLICATIONS: CARE OF THE VIGILING FAMILY

Family members have described what vigiling is and what this experience means to them. As a result, there are ways of caring for vigiling families that can be translated from research. The National Consensus Project for Quality Palliative Care developed specialized domains of care for patients and families during end of life. The domains include structures and processes; physical, psychological, social, spiritual, cultural, ethical, and legal aspects of care; and care of patient and family at end of life.[41] The vigil research extracted from this literature review has been synthesized, organized, and presented within this theoretical framework, to provide a guide to care for vigiling families (**Box 1**).

Box 1
Eight domains of care for vigiling families

Structures and Processes

- Promotion of interdisciplinary plan of care and documentation
- Assure education and training of direct staff on end-of-life care
- Facilitate communication between family members and staff
- Provide education on systems and processes at end of life
- Development of quality indicators for palliative nursing care
- Development of policy related to the family vigil experience

Physical Aspects of Care

- Provide comfort to patient and family
- Pain and symptom management for dying family member
- Encourage physical contact and communication with dying patient
- Provide nourishment and fluids to family

- Provide adequate and comfortable seating
- Provide pillows and blankets for night vigilers

Psychological and Psychiatric Aspects of Care

- Establish nurse–family relationship
- Assess awareness and acknowledge impending loss
- Assess of emotional needs of family
- Provide psychological preparation for death
- Allow for family locus of control
- Provide emotional support to family
- Assess anticipatory grief
- Assess bereavement risk
- Educate on bereavement services
- Make referrals for complicated grief

Social Aspects of Care

- Provide a private family space
- Provide homelike environment with personal belongings
- Open visitation hours: provide for uninterrupted family time
- Allow for family gathering and togetherness for vigil
- Balance need for private time for each family member
- Honor patient wishes for invited and uninvited guests
- Be present with patients and families as needed
- Make families aware you are close when you are not present
- Provide assessment and make referrals as needed to social work

Spiritual, Religious, and Existential Aspects of Care

- Offering of self and presence in the moment
- Listening and therapeutic communication
- Early assessment for spiritual distress
- Early assessment of need for pastoral care and clergy
- Assess family's spiritual beliefs regarding death
- Assess for music therapy referral
- Assess wishes regarding spiritual practices
- Provide family access to spiritual support
- Explore meaning of the lived experience of vigil keeping

Cultural Aspects of Care

- Provision of culturally competent staff
- Promote cultural curiosity among staff
- Provision of interpreter for effective communication
- Assess cultural beliefs and values of family
- Assess and honor culturally based rituals and practices
- Ongoing staff education on culture, beliefs, rituals, and practices

Care of the Patient and Family at End of Life

- Provide comprehensive and compassionate end-of-life care
- Provide information regarding progression of disease
- Educate on signs and symptoms of approaching death
- Provide normalization of dying process
- Offer prognostic time parameters if available
- Explore funeral planning/arrangements

Ethical and Legal Aspects of Care

- Establish health care proxy
- Establish advance directives
- Establish wishes regarding other treatments
- Support decisions regarding for or against life-prolonging measures
- Assess family for signs of ethical or moral dilemma
- Ensure referral to ethics committee as indicated

DISCUSSION

During the trajectory of life-threatening illness until the period of death, nurses fulfill the role of caregiver, advocate, and guide to patients and families throughout this transition. The role as caregiver provides nursing presence and the assurance that patient and family are the focus of care. The role as advocate provides resources to meet family needs, and the role as guide creates a peaceful environment for family gathering, providing information and support throughout the process of dying and death.[9] End-of-life research informs nurses that within the dying experience are opportunities to care for vigiling families with positive outcomes such as finding meaning through loss, family satisfaction, healing, growth, and transformation.[9,10,13]

ACKNOWLEDGMENTS

Acknowledgement and gratitude to Patricia Donohue-Porter, PhD, of Adelphi University and Lara Dhingra, PhD of MJHS Institute for Innovation in Palliative Care for their review and insights on this manuscript.

REFERENCES

1. Center for Disease Control and Prevention. Place of death, over time: United States, 1989, 1997, 2007. Available at: http://www.cdc.gov/nchs/data/hus/2010/fig33.pdf. Accessed March 20, 2016.
2. Doka K. Re-creating meaning in the face of illness. In: Rando T, editor. Clinical dimensions of anticipatory mourning: theory and practice in working with the dying, their loved ones, and their caregivers. Champaign (IL): Research Press; 2000. p. 103–13.
3. Glaser B, Strauss A. Awareness of dying. New Brunswick (NJ): Adline Transaction; 1965.
4. Cincotta N. The end of life at the beginning of life: working with dying children and their families. In: Berzoff J, Silverman P, editors. Living with dying: a handbook for

end of life healthcare practitioners. New York: Columbia University Press; 2004. p. 273–96.

5. Hottensen D. Anticipatory grief in patients with cancer. Clin J Oncol Nurs 2010; 14(1):106–9.

6. Rando T. Clinical dimensions of anticipatory mourning: theory and practice in working with the dying and their loved ones, and their caregivers. Champaign (IL): Research Press; 2000.

7. Worden W. Grief counseling and grief therapy. New York: Springer; 2002.

8. Davies B. Anticipatory mourning and the transition of fading away. In: Rando TA, editor. Clinical dimensions of anticipatory mourning. Champaign (IL): Research Press; 2000. p. 139–46.

9. Zerwekh JV. Nursing care at the end of life: palliative care for patients and families. Philadelphia: Davis; 2006.

10. Ferrell B, Coyle N. The nature of suffering and the goals of nursing. New York: Oxford University Press; 2008.

11. Ferrell B, Smith S, Juarez G, et al. Meaning of illness and spirituality in ovarian cancer survivors. Oncol Nurs Forum 2003;30(2):249–57.

12. Hung-Ru L, Bauer SM. Psycho-spiritual well-being in patients with advanced cancer. J Adv Nurs 2003;44(1):69–80.

13. Okun B, Nowinski J. Saying goodbye: how families can find renewal through loss. New York; Berkeley (CA): Harvard Health Publications; 2011. p. 27–73.

14. Field MJ, Cassel C, editors. Approaching death: improving end of life. Washington, DC: National Academies Press; 1997.

15. Meier D, Isaacs S, Hughes R. Palliative care. San Francisco (CA): Jossey-Bass; 2010.

16. Germino B, McCorkle R. Acknowledged awareness of life-threatening illness. Int J Nurs Stud 1985;22(1):33–44.

17. Reed PG. Spiritually and well-being in terminally ill hospitalized adults. Res Nurs Health 1987;10(3):335–44.

18. Ferrell B, Grant M, Virani R. Strengthening nursing education to improve end of life care. Nurs Outlook 1999;47(2):252–6.

19. Jeffers S. Nurse Faculty perceptions of end-of-life education in the clinical setting: a phenomenologic perspective. Ann Arbor (MI): Proquest Dissertations; 2011.

20. Institute of Medicine. Dying in America: improving quality and honoring individual preferences nearing the end of life. Washington, DC: National Academy Press; 2015.

21. Meleis A, editor. Transitions theory: middle range and situation-specific theories in nursing research and practice. New York: Springer; 2010. p. 1–23.

22. Larkin PJ, De Casterle LP, Schotsmans BD. Transition towards end of life in palliative care: exploration of its meaning for advanced cancer patients in Europe. In: Meleis AI, editor. Transitions theory: middle-range and situation-specific theories in nursing research. New York: Springer; 2010. p. 396–409.

23. Kastenbaum RJ. Death, society, and human experience. Boston: Allyn & Bacon; 2000.

24. Kastenbaum RJ. On our way: the final passage through life and death. Berkeley (CA): University of California Press; 2007.

25. Kuisle KA. (2002). Vigil: a psychological perspective. Unpublished doctoral dissertation. Union Institute and University Graduate College. Retrieved from: Proquest Dissertations and Theses database, (UMI No. 3052398), 2002.

26. Phillips PG, Reed LR. Into the abyss of someone else's dying: the voice of the end-of-life caregiver. Clin Nurs Res 2009;18(1):80–97.
27. Lindemann E. The symptomatology and management of acute grief. Am J Psychiatry 1944;101(1):141–8.
28. Meiers S, Brauer D. Existential caring in the family health experience: a proposed conceptualization. Scand J Caring Sci 2008;22(3):110–7.
29. Vigil. Oxford Dictionary. Available at: oxforddictionaries.com/us/definition/American-English/vigil. Accessed January 30, 2016.
30. Meyer G. The art of watching out: vigilance in women who have migraine headaches. Qual Health Res 2002;12(9):1220–34.
31. Carr J. Vigilance as a caring expression and Leininger's theory of cultural care, diversity, and universality. Nurs Sci Q 1998;11(1):74–8.
32. Mahoney D, Jones R, Coon D, et al. The caregiver vigilance scale: application and validation in the resources for enhancing Alzheimer's caregiver health (REACH) project. Am J Alzheimers Dis Other Demen 2003;18:39–48.
33. Eggenberger S, Krumweide N, Meiers S, et al. Family caring strategies in neutropenia. Clin J Oncol Nurs 2004;16:617–21.
34. Krumwiede N, Meiers S, Eggenberger S, et al. Turbulent waiting: rural families experiencing chemotherapy-induced neutropenia. Oncol Nurs Forum 2004;31(6):1142–5.
35. Morse JM, O'Brien B. Preserving self: from victim, to patient, to disabled person. J Adv Nurs 1995;21(2):886–96.
36. Fridh I, Forberg A, Bergbom I. Close relative's experiences of caring and of the physical environment when a family member dies in ICU. Intensive Crit Care Nurs 2008;25:111–9.
37. Read T, Wuest J. Daughters caring for dying parents: a process of relinquishing. Qual Health Res 2007;17(7):932–44.
38. Williams B, Amos-Bailey F, Woodby L, et al. A room full of chairs around his bed: being present at the death of a family member in veteran's affairs medical centers. Omega (Westport) 2013;66(3):231–63.
39. Bell C. Ritual: perspectives and dimension. New York: Oxford; 1997.
40. van Gennep A. The rites of passage. Chicago: University of Chicago Press; 1960.
41. Dahlin C. The National Consensus Project for Quality Palliative Care: clinical practice guidelines for quality palliative care. 3rd Edition. 2013.

Rituals at End-of-Life

James C. Pace, PhD, MDiv, APRN, BC, FAANP, FAAN[a],*,
Tyree S. Mobley, BS, RN[b]

KEYWORDS

- Rituals • Rites • Ceremonies • End-of-life • Deathbed • Child death • Perinatal loss
- Sacraments

KEY POINTS

- Rituals include activities that involve gestures, words, and objects performed in selected places and sequences of time.
- Rituals at end of life (EOL) enhance the quality of life and support those dying and the living who grieve.
- Rituals at EOL contribute to the strength, capacity, and health of professional providers who cope with multiple death events.
- Rituals help the living to create continuing bonds with those dying, help with coping skills by increasing feelings of control and power, and assist with the finding of meaning in life.

BACKGROUND: RITUALS AT END OF LIFE REFLECT, APPRECIATE, AND HONOR LIFE

One of the major themes to emerge from reports of dying patients and their surviving family members is the extreme importance of rituals at EOL.[1–5] A ritual has been defined as a sequence of activities involving gestures, words, and objects performed in a specific place and sequence of time.[6] Rituals help participants to cross from their present situation to another and, therefore, describe an important change in status.[5] Rituals encase memories and link the past with the present.[7,8] Rituals are an antidote to powerlessness.[9] Rituals help patients find meaning in life, enter into a comfort zone, create memories that confirm life accomplishments, assuage a sense of loss, and create a roadmap for dying "the right way."[1,2,10,11] Rituals address the need to comprehend existence in a meaningful way, establish relationships, attach order, and posit a place in the wonder and the mystery of life.[8,11] Rituals can help the dying focus on living rather than the processes of dying, giving richer meaning to each day of life.[1] The meaning of rituals for the dying not only are important to patients but also to family members and caregivers.[1,8] Rituals can involve religious themes and the use of material objects (such as rosary beads); and for those who

Disclosures: No disclosures.
[a] NYU Rory Meyers College of Nursing, 433 First Avenue, New York, NY 10010, USA;
[b] Stroudsburg, PA, USA
* Corresponding author.
E-mail address: jcp12@nyu.edu

claim no religious beliefs, rituals become an important substitute (such as the observance of a holiday, cooking special meals, or creating a legacy book). The search for meaning that can be found in rituals does not need to be overtly philosophic or religious on the grand scale; the search can be circumscribed, such as, "What has been the importance of my life for my family?" Rituals are multidimensional; they include any ceremony, rite, procedure, or behavior that is performed in a set manner. Rituals can be simple or complex, formal or informal, cultural or religious, instructive or constructive, private or public, individual or corporate, one-time or repetitive, passive or active, or rigid or flexible.[3,7,11]

Rituals allow expressing emotions; feeling secure in the midst of chaos; ordering experiences outside our control; reinforcing group ties; communicating thoughts, ideas, and feelings; reinforcing values; entering into a change of status; marking a rite of passage; expressing grief; articulating meaning and purpose; and transforming what is ordinary into the extraordinary, sacred, and holy.[7]

THE SPIRITUAL AND RELIGIOUS IMPORTANCE OF RITUAL(S)

Life-threatening illness is a crisis time for many who are laden with medical, psychological, social, and family ramifications.[4] As people approach death, there is also the distinct possibility for a spiritual crisis.[12] Spirituality is a human need and people have a variety of ways in which they find, or fail to find, transcendent meaning in the world around them.[13] The religious and spiritual realms can be hard to define, differentiate, and distinguish because they are often elusive concepts and carry many meanings. The National Consensus Project for Quality Palliative Care identifies spirituality as an essential domain of care.[14,15] Ferrell and Borneman[15] state that quality care for patients and families is not possible without quality spiritual care. For the purpose of this article, definitions of key terms follow.[12,16]

Spirituality

Spirituality is personal, individual and eclectic and reflects one's deep inner essence. Spirituality is a search for meaning; it is often ineffable and includes what is considered valued, important, and memorable. Spiritual practices may include prayer and the use of ritual.

Religion

Religion serves to delineate the beliefs that are shared by a group or a community of faith. Religion often specifies the ways that individuals or groups are to behave or act and may teach about some form of continuity after death. Religious rituals provide comfort to the bereaved in communal practices.[13,17]

Spirituality may be shaped by religious beliefs and is also impacted by cultural perspective and personal experiences during a lifetime. When confronting life-threatening illness, dying, and death, spiritual and religious beliefs may be called into question. Both religion and spirituality can play a key role in helping to make sense of illness, find strength, and create meaning.[18] The realms of spirit and belief can reduce feelings of fear and minimize uncertainty.[12,18] Many individuals benefit from the social support and pastoral care provided by the ministries of chaplains, clergy, spiritual advisors, and faith communities. Religious and spiritual factors may have positive effects on health, including enhanced positive coping skills, enhanced self-esteem, and increased feelings of control, hope, and strength.[12,19] Religious and spiritual factors may also have detrimental effects, including increased death anxiety, guilt, and fear to the point that health may be further compromised.[12,19] Health care professionals have long realized that the patient/family spiritual and religious beliefs have an impact on health care outcomes.[19] Rituals are drawn from religious and/or spiritual beliefs/practices that offer patients and their family member(s) a newfound sense of meaning, purpose, and comfort.[12] Health care professionals who have knowledge of the range of possibilities for rituals at EOL and their practical applications are better able to serve the needs of their patients and families.

MEANINGFUL RITUALS AT MISCARRIAGE, STILLBIRTH, AND NEWBORN DEATH

Perinatal loss is defined as "…an unwanted end of pregnancy during 40 weeks of gestation (through miscarriage or stillbirth) or during the first 28 days of life (the neonatal period)."[3] Rituals for grieving the life-never-lived of a stillborn child or a child who dies soon after birth are important for all those who attempt to adjust to life without their baby.[20] Parent(s) and siblings of a perinatal loss who will not have opportunities to watch their baby grow need opportunities to say goodbye and remember. Such rituals are often neglected due to time constraints, veiled communication patterns, lack of direction, feeling rushed by family or staff, believing that time spent with the dead is moribund or unnatural, or confusion as to what to do next.[20] Sadly, "most stillborn babies are disposed of without any recognition or ritual."[21] Parents find comfort in rituals; they report an intense yearning to hold, touch, rock, and care for their child. One important ritual involves 3 steps: see, hold, and name[10]—seeing the baby and holding the baby create memories for a lifetime; knowing and naming the child during this important time can be healing. Counting fingers and toes, ears, arms, legs, becomes important, because any sense of normalcy is comforting. Some parents choose to bathe the child.

A picture is worth a lifetime of memory; it becomes a treasured keepsake.[20] A hospital can arrange for professional pictures to be taken or parents can use cellphones or personal cameras. When parents of a child who died in a hospital were asked what they wished they could have done differently, they replied that they wished they had spent more time with their baby, held their baby longer, kissed their baby more, took time to love their baby. Seeing and holding are important actions; parents who have been interviewed years later stated how thankful they were that they took the time to remember how the baby felt and looked, observing every freckle and every part.[10] If there are no remains to bury, a specific ritual that can be implemented is to take a photograph of the child's hand (from either a photo or scan), cutting it out, and placing it in an outline of a picture of the parent(s) hand(s). Both can then be buried together and prayers can be said at the burial site.[22] Some parents found it helpful to write letters to their child and make copies to keep, the originals being buried with the child. Some parents have taken the child's ashes and buried them in their yard set apart with a specially carved marker or stone; some burn a candle beside the marker on the anniversary of birth/death.[20] Finally, parents of infants who die often appreciate being unburdened at some point after the loss. Being told that they did not cause the death relieves them of misplaced feelings of guilt that they somehow (almost always mistakenly) attribute to self or to a partner.[23] An example of an unburdening ritual is in **Box 1**.

Likewise, members of the health care team often benefit from a kind word or a pastoral response from a colleague/peer who seeks to unburden them as well. A comment such as, "I would have done exactly the same things that you did. You did not miss anything, and you did everything you could have done." Unburdening parents and staff of misplaced guilt is a ritual that provides reassurance, relief, and release.[23]

> **Box 1**
> **A Ritual of Unburdening**
>
> I'm so sorry that this happened, but it did not happen because of anything you did or did not do. This is absolutely not either of your faults. Many parents, especially moms, think it's somehow their fault when their newborn dies. It's clearly not true here. If you had done something to cause this, I would tell you so that it wouldn't happen again. But you did not cause this and you couldn't have prevented it.
>
> *From* Mercurio MR. Rituals of Unburdening. Hastings Cent Rep 2008;38(2):8–9.

THE MALE PERSPECTIVE OF PERINATAL LOSS

The impact of perinatal loss on the male partners of women who have lost a child has been largely overlooked.[24] Such losses can be devastating to the male's partner, and yet he may feel that culture dictated that he has to discount the loss (thereby taking attention away from the father) and devote significant attention to support the mother both immediately and over a sustained period of time.[24] Several recurring themes have been associated with male loss, including self-blame, loss of identity, the need to appear strong, feelings of marginalization and neglect, and the need to hide feelings of grief and anger.[24] Men may seek the permission of others to express their own needs and to feel normal with such a request. Lasker and Toedter[25] report that men are at risk of developing a chronic grief response to pregnancy loss because they do not receive the support they need to effectively deal with the loss. Many men blame themselves for things, such as not taking their partner to a medical provider sooner, not listening to complaints made by their partner, ignoring potential health care needs of their partner, or feeling that staff members blamed them for the loss. Men found their own needs validated when they were allowed the opportunity to bury the remains, to be listed on any documents that pertain to the death (eg, the death certificate), to express such emotions as crying, to share the role of telling others (rather than bearing the entire responsibility for the communication of the loss to others), to share the role of planning a funeral with family members, and to have specially designated staff members listen and devote attention to the man after the death event (independently of the mother). Fathers also found it important to be given the opportunity to hold the dead child and have their own photographs of the deceased, locks of hair, and an article of clothing or blanket. People who call the home to express condolences should actively ask how the male partner is doing, not just inquire of the mother's status. Men should avail themselves of self-help and support groups tailored to their gender where, with others who have experienced similar events and emotions, they can share their interpretations and feelings. Such groups have organized community memorial services where names are entered into a memorial book of remembrance, flowers are placed in a common vase, candles are lit, poems are said, and songs sung. Such rituals sanction grief, recognize sorrow, and the importance/value of those lost.[24] When institutions have an annual communal service for bereaved parents, the male partner should be individually invited (along with their partner). Men also felt validated when their identity was confirmed as that of being the father.[24]

RITUALS IN THE CRITICAL CARE SETTING

Critical care settings are by their nature places where lives are meant to be saved. Heroic measures are actively engaged to preserve life, sometimes seemingly at all costs.[26] During highly stressful episodes in these settings, there is often a lack of time for the planning and implementing rituals that might allow for time for taking leave of someone near death. Death sometimes is associated with human failure. Often, a nurse is aware of the dying event and wants to be able to communicate this to the dying patient as well as to the family/friends but is so caught up with the demands of care delivery that such moral courage is sidetracked by practical concerns and the practical provision of as much comfort as is possible.[26] During such events, it is important for staff to give space and time for survivors who want to be present after the death. The body needs to be appropriate prepared, equipment removed when possible, and the site made as welcoming as possible. Although family should be given time alone with the deceased, staff need to be attentive to the needs of family members who may have intense grief reactions. Caring practices allow for touch and the vocalizations of love, sorrow, apologies, and even anger. Religious rituals conducted by pastoral care providers/clergy can be useful and necessary. Prayers of thanksgiving for a life short lived and the honoring of the deceased can be key components of such rituals (Appendix 1).

RITUALS IN THE EMERGENCY ROOM

In the emergency department, the injuries often overwhelm the capacity of the staff to repair and to heal.[27] Jonathan Bartels, a trauma nurse at the University of Virginia, described many such events, where, after the death is called, workers leave the emergency suite feeling defeated, often in emotional pain, and have to quickly turn their backs to the patient's now lifeless body and scramble to their next emergency. "I felt one thing missing was to ritualize or acknowledge what just happened in front of us," said Bartels.[28] After one particular death, a chaplain who was present asked all staff to stop for a moment so that a prayer could be said before leaving the room. It was at that moment that Bartels knew what he needed to do. With the permission and guidance of his nursing administrators, Bartels created "the pause," where staff members stop what they are doing immediately after the death is called and think about the patient as an individual before resuming their work. Bartels states that the pause gives a moment of reverence to the death event and has the capacity to reframe potential feelings of being defeated by death. The pause shows respect and honor for the dead while helping to improve the mindset of the health care providers who gather together in mutual support and understanding. A typical pause lasts anywhere from 45 to 60 seconds. Some of those gathered around the table are known to pray whereas others silently reflect on the life of the individual and his/her family.

The death of a child in the emergency department is always difficult. In the emergency department, the occurrence of such an event is unplanned, rushed, anxiety producing, and filled with a magnitude of tragedy.[29] In addition to all the complexities of the compassionate care being rendered, there are multiple possible responsibilities: when to withdraw no longer beneficial medical interventions; organ procurement discussions; notification of security, chaplain, and medical examiner; consents for postmortem examinations and benefit of autopsy; child protective services; preservation of evidence; and when to allow/encourage family presence, to name only a few. Childhood death (age younger than 18) is not an expected part of life and is uncommon.[29] Providers who are used to "the routinization of disaster" may not be in the best situation to provide kind, empathetic, and genuinely calm care and responses to a family.[30] Yet, communication skills and family involvement in the last moments of life are what families remember.[29] How to relay difficult information (ie, bad news) may be one of the most important EOL rituals possible to the health care team.[31] Family presence during resuscitation in the patient care area has received widespread endorsement because resuscitation because it allows family access to rituals that may involve the recitation of prayers or simply to reach out, touch, and/or hold a hand.[32,33] Families find such activities helpful and staff reported no disruption in care.[34] When family members cannot arrive to the emergency setting prior to the death event, an alternative to prolonging a futile resuscitation attempt is to assign a staff member to serve as a surrogate family member whose role it is to be with the child at all times until family arrive. The surrogate can then discuss all that was done to care for the child and to assure family that their child was never left alone.[29] Such postmortem communication by staff members allows for memory making on the part of the family, easing them into a healthier sense of bereavement. Parents viewed such staff members as "keepers of the memory" of their child. Small gestures of condolence, such as cards, phone calls, texts, and e-mails, have profound and positive effects on surviving family.[29] Allowing family members to say their good-byes to the deceased child in whatever ways is valuable to them is encouraged because it is critical to the well-being of the bereaved family. It is also helpful to ask if there are any rituals involved in the aftercare of the deceased that may involve religious belief; for example, it may not be acceptable for the body of the deceased to be handled or cared for by someone of the opposite gender. It may be helpful to ask, "Does your family culture or faith tradition give you guidance about what should happen after death? We would like to support you in that if we can."[29]

RITUALS ASSOCIATED WITH THE UNFOUND (THE MISSING)

Perhaps one of the most difficult types of human loss occurs when the body of the deceased cannot be found. In such situations, many find that they do not have the benefit of a traditional ritual of death (ie, a funeral or memorial service). The funeral is most often the event whereby the family marks the official beginning of a period of mourning and finding a sense of spiritual healing after death.[35] When there is no funeral and no remains to focus on, for many, the loss become incomprehensible because there is no chance to say good-bye or to complete unfinished business. Without the presence of a body, death can be unbelievable and difficult to accept; the bereaved may become locked or frozen in the hope that the lost will be found living and well. Boss[36] terms this phenomenon, "ambiguous loss" – without verification of a missing person's status, there is uncertainty, anxiety, confusion, and immobilization. With ambiguous loss, new roles cannot be entered into completely (widowhood or orphanhood, for examples).

Those mourning the unfound can be helped by referral to a grief counselor or mental health professional. The goal is to help an individual/family to accept the reality of the loss, allow the pain of grief, and adjust to a reality where the loved one is missing.[35] Active listening to the telling of stories and events is extremely important. Active listening should be done with patience, and responses should be authentic, without raising false hopes and expectations. Working through feelings of guilt and being open to the venting of anger are sound interventions that facilitate communication and the expression of emotion/feelings. The individual/family can be encouraged to hold a funeral or a memorial service that provides them with communal support. Such events are highly symbolic and meaningful; a treasured picture of the deceased might be a prominent display. Later, key articles of clothing (eg, a suit or formal dress) can be buried in a suitable location. The mourners are supported in their pain and uncertainty and are assured that their feelings are not due to something that they either did or did not do. The mourner is on a difficult journey to find meaning and is in a situation that stems from the total loss of control and the anguish of simply not knowing.

HONORING CEREMONIES

The Institute of Medicine has reported that advanced technology and extraordinary procedures have rendered death a medical event shaped by societal and cultural expectations. Death, more often than not, occurs in hospitals and often without family and friends present. What is studied and what is published about the culture of dying often describes only what leads up to the time of death itself. Little is written about the time after death and how nurses render care and perceive how much their actions have an impact on the environment around them, to include the culture of postmortem care. In the few initial studies that are available concerning the impact of honoring ceremonies that take place after a death occurs and their impact on staff members, there seems to be improved staff satisfaction and a renewed sense of dedication.[37] Honoring ceremonies provide staff and family with a sense of closure allowing for movement forward.[37] In addition, there is an abiding bond that forms between staff and family that would not be present if such a ceremony did not take place. The major impact of an honoring ceremony is that it eases the transition through death and the immediate time period that follows the death event. The ceremony may be simple in approach: it may be a reading of a scripted poem or statement with all gathered around the deceased (when possible). The deceased is remembered and the staff are commended for their care and there is release to go forth to the next task/assignment.[22,37] An example of a brief ritual that honors the deceased as well as providing a means for the staff to rededicate themselves to their work is in **Box 2**.

The deceased is remembered as well as the surviving family. Such a ceremony not only increases the depth and feeling of compassion offered by all present but also gives courage to move on.[22,37]

The Department of Veterans Affairs has instituted policies and procedures for "Honoring Deceased Veterans at Time of In-Hospital Death."[38] The honoring ceremony consists of draping the gurney that bears the veteran's remains with a service flag (not the American flag). The service flag is an official banner authorized by the Department of Defense to honor men and women who serve in the Armed Forces. The service flag–draped gurney is taken from the unit to the morgue, and, whenever possible, staff line the route for a moment of silence as the gurney makes its way to the morgue. Once the remains have been transported to the morgue, an American flag is placed on the bedside table of the deceased veteran and the table is placed in the doorway. The flag remains in place until the room is needed for the next patient.

At a hospice in California, an honoring ceremony includes the following rituals. When the mortician arrives to claim the body, it is properly shrouded, placed on the gurney, and removed to a specially constructed garden outside. There, all staff are invited to gather and time is devoted to stories, song, remembrances, or simply a time for silence; the remains are then sprinkled with flower petals (D. Wholihan, personal communication, 2016).

Box 2
Closing ritual at the bedside of the deceased

I thank everyone here for your compassionate care and your efforts to do everything possible for (*name of patient*). Let us take a moment in silence to acknowledge our sorrow at (*his/her*) death and to remember the family at their time of loss. Let us be reminded constantly of the honor and the wonder of the work that we do.

From Barkas D, Voigtritter S, Shynk T. Compassion doesn't end when the heart stops: nurse's perceptions of honoring ceremony at end-of-life. Clinical Nurse Specialist 2014;28(2):E11

The most widely known honoring ceremony is the funeral. There are several purposes of the funeral: it is a socially acceptable form of communal gathering that allows for group support; it allows those present to validate the life and the significance of the deceased; it confirms the actuality of the death; it gives meaning to the power of memory in and through active, stimulating expression; and, for some, allows for the religious themes of hope and vision of the life eternal.[35,39] Such rituals not only are about letting go of the physicality of the deceased and connecting in a more spiritual way but also become a time when leave can be taken and successful grieving can begin. In this new place, and supported by others, a new found strength is often found, allowing moving on.

LEGACY MAKING: PRESERVING MEMORIES

Legacy gifts/tokens are beneficial to survivors of the death of a loved one.[3,40] Any such gift can be placed in a memory box that is given to, created for, or preserved by the survivor.

Postmortem Photography

Photographs (taken with the permission of the survivors) may have increased value over succeeding years.[40,41] Photographed images can have a positive value in coming to successful terms with grief and acknowledging the reality of death.[41,42]

Molds, Inks, Castings, and Material Objects (the Importance of a Memento)

Art therapy rituals include hand and foot molds made out of model magic clay or plaster gauze and handprints and footprints using inkless wipes and papers. Mementos, such as a lock of hair, a hospital band, scrapbooks of cards and letters, balloons, hair accessories, jewelry, dried flowers, shoes, clothing, and blanket(s), can be vital component parts of the memory box.[40,42] Mementos, such as those described, allow opportunities to find peace, to remember ("I will never forget"), to say goodbye to loved ones, and to address the significance of existence.[42]

Social Media

A personal Facebook account can be turned into a memorialized account on the request of friends and family, with documentation of an obituary or other documentation about the death. To the site, pictures can be posted as can communications with the deceased. A Facebook account can be an evolving eulogy that gives form to multiple expressions of love and devotion.[43]

MAINTAINING (CONTINUING) BONDS: POSTDEATH ENCOUNTERS

Some family members are able to maintain a continuing relationship with their deceased loved one through visualization, imagination, and dreams.[40] Visualization may take the form of imagining how a child has grown or how an adult might have aged. Some seek advice, guidance, and comfort from the spirit of the deceased and report much comfort from these ongoing relationships.[40] Some believe that the spirit of their deceased loved one has become their guardian angel and can lend divine assistance. These examples of maintaining bonds and the associated rituals behind them reveal how unique and multidimensional the effects of healing can be.

The bereaved often report postdeath encounters: seeing, hearing, or feeling the presence of the deceased.[44] Some term these experiences, *idionecrophanies* or *paranormal* or *extraordinary postdeath contacts or experiences*, often occurring soon after death but sometimes longer, even years.[45] Auditory and visual apparitions are the most frequently reported postdeath contacts, followed by imperceptible presence.[44,46] A majority of individuals report these as pleasant and comforting and leading to a sense of connection with the deceased and to a newfound sense of closure. Many believe that such experiences demonstrate that loving relationships have the power to transcend death.[47] For most, contact with deceased helps with their bereavement responses, reducing unresolved feelings of loss, grief, guilt, and sadness and helping to provide hope, peace, and the ability to move forward.[44] Postdeath encounters are best discussed with those who remain nonjudgmental and who are interested in helping the bereaved find meaning in the encounter. Many are unwilling to discuss their encounters for fear of being ridiculed or being diagnosed with mental illness.[44] Rituals that allow strategies for maintaining bonds with the deceased include[47]

- Imagined interactions and internal dialogues
- Verbal communications (to include prayer)
- Remembering and recording (diary) memories and dreams
- Celebrating memorials and holding anniversary celebrations
- Having a purposed discussion with a friend/relative about the deceased
- Reviewing a detailed life story of the person who has died

Health care professionals do well to focus on the therapeutic effects of continuing bond encounters because such experiences can bring healing, notions of wholeness, connectedness, and transcendence.[44,47]

RITUAL AT END OF LIFE AS SACRAMENT
Baptism

The baptism of newborns as well as the baptism of adults occurs frequently at EOL scenarios and is a significantly important event, even in the life a provider who may not believe.[48] Admittedly, baptism is a uniquely Christian event in the lives of those who believe in its place and power. Many believe baptism to be an outward sign of a significant spiritual change in the lives of those who believe. Often it is difficult for nursing staff to find a pastoral care provider/clergy person to officiate at a baptism, particularly when there is urgency or during late nights, holidays, or weekends. In the life of believers, baptism might assure that the newly baptized is forgiven and will forever be with God in eternity.[48] "Baptizing a baby may be the family and baby's only opportunity to celebrate God's grace on this earth."[48] In the case of an emergency, a nurse can validly baptize, using the example format in Appendix 2.

Marriage

Health care professionals are often asked to assist with plans for a quickly arranged marriage ceremony at the bedside involving a patient who is near death. For example, despite a terminal cancer diagnosis, a bride can be radiant, dressed in scarf and headpiece and with carefully applied make-up by loving family members. The ceremony can serve as a keystone event that brings together family, providers, case managers, social workers, chaplains, and staff.

The pastoral care department can lend ready assistance with legal details and how to construct a liturgy of marriage that is congruent with patient and family values. Depending on the state, state laws recognize who can legally officiate at marriage ceremonies to include members of the clergy, a judge, court clerk, and justices of the peace. In some states, all of these must be officially certified or licensed by the state before they can officiate at a marriage. Some states allow other persons to apply for permission to become a deputy commissioner of marriage – this status grants authority that is valid for 1 day – who thus can officiate at a marriage for family/friend.[49] Bedside marriage ceremonies can assist the newly married to achieve a new level of comfort, allowing them to finally rest easy.[50]

Anointing with Oil

The anointing of the sick with oil bears many titles: last rites, anointing, sacrament of the sick, blessing of the sick, ministry of healing, and extreme unction.[11,51] Usually, the rite is conducted in an orderly format by a priest or an ordained representative. Theologically, the rite no longer specifically marks the EOL (active dying) but rather the start of living with illness and all manner of health outcomes that may lie ahead. The anointing marks an individual's belief in the eternal and provides strength, courage, forgiveness, and God's never-failing support of the sick and the dying.[51]

RITUAL DRAMA: MUSIC THERAPY AT THE BEDSIDE

Ritual dramas at EOL include any and all variations of performances (which can be live or recorded) that involve a performer, any gathered caregivers, and the person who is near death. Such performances bring out the essential nature of liminality, a key characteristic involved in all rituals. Liminality assumes that, within the ritual itself, there is some point of transition for the person to whom the ritual is addressed. The liminal state nurtures a transition point that marks the success of the ritual, and the patient successfully moves into a new understanding of the current state. There is every possibility for the transformation into a more peaceful state marked by the meaning of newfound awareness. The performance is meant to create a possibility for an eased transition in which each participant invests the experience with evolving meaning. Thus, music therapy and music at the bedside offer an unfolding drama where participants join in a process that brings a successful transition point to the loved one.[52] Music allows shifting in and out of melodies, rhythms, harmonies, and timbres to meet the need of the situation. The 3 stages of ritual drama (through music) are parting/separation, liminality, and reintegration. These 3 stages have also been termed, *rite of passage ritual structures*.[11] Music allows separating from a previous position and traveling into the liminal, a place of transition. An old world view gives way to a new. A music therapist facilitates the transition and transformation. With reintegration, the ritual passenger is reintroduced into life and living in a new position and with new identities in place (a postlife construct).[52] Ritual drama allows participants an intersubjective process that leads to healing and wellness. "Music is a culturally informed medium that shapes to the cultural, spiritual, and lived traditions that conceive and perform it."[52] Its purpose is to move those who enter into a more peaceful point of transition and the new awareness that follows.

COLLECTIVE RESPONSES TO DEATH

Public expressions of grief and trauma can be given collective expression. Public memorials can be created/situated where individuals or groups of people can bring such things as teddy bears, toys, flowers, candles, votives, written notes, wreaths, and religious articles (such as crucifixes and rosaries). These items serve as icons of hope and coping.[53] Public spiritual shrines allow for collective expressions of grief and discussions and serve as a locations where collective suffering can be shared and even welcomed.[53] Often the site of a traumatic event can be recognized with an engraved plaque to serve as a permanent reminder of death. Such places constitute a death system, where society is given a means to respond to a collective or public death as well as to the death of a private individual. Such places allow for the expression of unresolved grief, altruism, and solidarity and provide new forums for sharing memories, expressing empathy and compassion. Creating rituals or simply allowing them to happen at such sites provides individuals with a means to find closure, create meaning around experiences with loss, and build a sense of belonging to a community and society.

VARIOUS OTHER RITUALS

- Burning a pink candle all day on Christmas Day to represent the presence of a lost one
- Visiting the graveside annually on the date of death and doing a crayon rub of the gravestone
- Planting a tree/shrub to commemorate a life
- Donating a tangible object that commemorates a life while being enjoyed by others (a park bench); naming a classroom space
- Cleansing of guilt: the asking of forgiveness at the graveside
- Donating flowers/sanctuary candles at church in honor of the dead
- The birthday party: parent(s) and loved ones can celebrate the birth of a child in a critical care or hospice setting with all the trappings of a birthday party: banners, cards, singing, birthday hats. The only thing out of the ordinary with such a party is that it might occur way too early for it to be the first birthday party and far too early for it to be the last. Families can face the death of a child by first celebrating the life of the child. The family can be clearly aware of what is happening but choose to commemorate what was rather than what will be. They celebrate a childhood ritual to celebrate a small amount of time available. Despite the shortness of life, there can be love and devotion and the value of every minute. Mourning and grief can be accompanied by joy and celebration, too.[54]

  Likewise, a birthday party before its time can be held for a person of any age and at any time. Birthday parties are considered a normal happy life event that supports the person dying, the family, and others in and through their participation.[55] During the event, there can be a specific time for the saying of "goodbye."
- Penitential psalms or psalms of confession: Psalms 6, 32, 38, 51, 102, 130, and 143
- Intercessory prayer: the prayers of others that are said (or thought) for the well-being of another offer friends and family members tangible things to say and do. Prayer is a way of coping for many and has been found to lower stress and promote a sense of peace.[51] Prayer can also entail words, silences, and images that resonate deep within and that heal.[56]
- It is recommended that children attend the visitation, funeral, and burial rituals (when held) of a deceased parent; although the death of a parent can be a traumatic event for children, attending death-related rituals has been shown to provide children with a perceived supportive community and a means from which children can draw comfort and bid their final goodbyes.[57]
- A leave-taking ritual at the bedside: often family members who gather at the bedside of the dying do not know what to do or what to say, especially in critical care situations where their loved one may be intubated, in a coma, and unable to talk and converse with family. In such situations, the following 5-step ritual may be important to describe:
  ○ Recount a happy, fulfilling, pleasant memory in your shared lives (the value of reminiscence that sets a positive tone).

- State that you forgive the patient of all harms and unpleasantries (acts of commission or omission) that occurred in the past.
- Ask personal forgiveness for any harms and unpleasantries done to the family member.
- Tell the patient that you love him/her.
- Say "good-bye" (one of the most frequent regrets of the living: "If only I had been able to say goodbye!").[58]

END-OF-LIFE RITUALS AND THE NURSE

It is often the nurse who is the last to hold the hand of one who transitions from life to death. Nurses who deal with EOL extensively need self-care and the care of others to include peers and administrative staff. Nurses benefit from continued training on how to deliver bad news, care for emotionally distraught family members, and in understanding personal feelings and behaviors. Debriefing times/ceremonies for critical incidents can be helpful in defusing guilt feelings or feelings of inadequacy, even failure. There is a healing potential in conducting closing rituals at the bedside of the patient who has died that may be beneficial to staff, several of which are reviewed previously. What is important for nurses to remember is that it is easy, over time, to develop a thick armor to shield the self from experiencing overwhelming loss. The nurse is often fully in control of his/her emotions at the time of a patient's death. After the death, and during care of the body of the deceased, high levels of anxiety may be expressed by laughing, joking, having casual conversation, and depersonalizing the body. The major roles of the nurse in caring for a body after death are to carry out legal requirements, protect the body tissues, and discharge the body to the appropriate area for claim.[59] Nursing actions after death may include the closing of the eyelids, inserting dentures and closing the mouth, positioning the body in a natural state, removing all tubes, and preparing the body to be viewed. Dressings are best wrapped with circular gauze/bandage or held in place by paper tape to prevent damage to the skin and algor mortis (ie, lack of skin integrity due to decreased body temperature).[59] In preparing a room for a family's visit to a loved one who has died, the nurse transforms the space into a sacred space. The lights should be dimmed as much as possible, the room cleaned of all equipment, and water and tissues should be available to those who visit.

Religious-based traditions of the family should be honored when possible. When the patient is from the Jewish tradition, the care of the body and final rites are to be coordinated with both family and rabbi. If the nurse is not the designated person to deliver postmortem care, the nurse may supervise or educate others about the need for respect for the dead, obeying religious rituals and cultural norms, and the need for attention to the sacred space of the dying.[8,10] Informative and compassionate information can be offered to those who wonder if it is culturally correct to hold a dead infant, get into the bed of a loved one who has just died, or to kiss the lips of the recently deceased.

Nurses need to care for one another's collected grief needs as well. A team debriefing conducted by the clinical manager or the chaplain may be effective in allowing team members to express their thoughts in a safe zone that serves to validate, support, and restore.[60] Names for such debriefings include mentor support meeting, facilitated team processing, reflective practice activities, staff self-care, and co-creating ritual.[60] During such meetings, all voices are heard and respected. The main objective is to process the grief of the group. The timing of such meetings varies depending on how many deaths are encountered and the individual events of each death (traumatic, long-term patient death, beloved patient death, staff dedication to a particular

---

Box 3
A ritual of honor and rededication

Loving God, we come to you with our sadness, our grief, and together we acknowledge the difficulties of our work. Grant us your presence so that we might be strengthened and so that we might reach new understandings of what we do and how to do it better now and in days to come. Loving God, we ask for your energy, wisdom, and guidance as we dedicate ourselves to our work. Make this space one of healing: less pain, less suffering, and less despair. Restore us and be with us. May your blessings be known through our hands, our hearts, and our words. Let us now go in peace, surrounded by our friends and the support that we offer, one to another. Amen.

From Kobler K. Leaning in and holding on: team support with unexpected death. MCN Am J Matern Child Nurs 2014;39(3):148–54.

---

patient/family, and so forth). During such meetings, staff should also be educated on best practices in handling individual grief.[61] Such exercises include PRAM: take time to *P*ause, *R*eflect, *A*cknowledge, be *M*indful.[60] Staff are able to connect with the reality of experiences, learn from them, and acknowledge their importance. In clinical settings, there is often time for a chaplain to be present with staff and lead them in a clinical rededication/blessing of the work space (**Box 3**). Such rituals are useful for staff to recenter, rededicate, and move forward.

SUMMARY

Rituals at EOL have the potential to help the dying achieve comfort, support, and relief from guilt and anger and to feel nurtured and confident (**Box 4**).[51]

Rituals allow participants to separate from what is happening, transition to a new state, and then begin to live in a transformed way. Rituals at EOL help the living to reorganize, reorient, and construct new ways of living that allow for healthy bereavement, remembering, honoring, and memorializing the dead.[2] Rituals allow a certain sense of control in what can often be perceived as an out-of-control world.[10] Rituals allow the

---

Box 4
Summary of the importance of rituals at end of life

- Provides a forum where death is acknowledged and accepted as real
- Legitimizes grief and different styles of grieving
- Provides structure and stability at a time of great uncertainty or chaos
- Raises self-esteem
- Affords a safe place to express emotion or grieving issues, being time-limited
- Sets a climate for a potent honoring of the deceased
- Clarifies issues
- Promotes a positive sense of life direction or meaning
- Gives a sense of community with the inclusion of others
- Promotes congruency: body, mind and spirit
- Encourages follow-through with public statements of intention

From Reeves N. Death acceptance through ritual. Death Stud. 2011;35(5):408–19.

---

construction of structures that allow coping with losses. Health care professionals need to expand on their definition, understanding, and practice of ritual. Rituals transfer the ordinary into the extraordinary and the everyday into the sacred. Rituals help people to connect and to trust. Losses should neither be hidden nor unacknowledged but rather recognized, remembered, and held sacred. Sacred memories can be loving memorials rather than morbid reminders of grief. Rituals help family members and providers take courage to continue with their lives and the work they have been given to do.

REFERENCES

1. Cancer Network. Study of dying cancer patients reveals importance of rituals. Oncol News Int 2000;9(5):28–9. Available at: http://search.ebscohost.com/login.aspx?direct=true&db=rzh&AN=106908821&site=ehost-live. Accessed February 29, 2016.
2. Corso VM. Rituals that reflect and honor life. Death Stud 2009;33(3):287–91.
3. Côté-Arsenault D. Weaving babies lost in pregnancy into the fabric of the family. J Fam Nurs 2003;9(1):23–37, 15p.
4. Myers GE. Restoration or transformation? Choosing ritual strategies for end-of-life care. Mortality 2003;8(4):372–87.
5. Reeves N. Death acceptance through ritual. Death Stud 2011;35(5):408–19.
6. Bell C. Ritual: perspectives and dimension. New York: Oxford; 1997.
7. Vande Kieft D. Rituals (blessings) for the dying time [handout]. Snohomish (WA): Providence Hospice of Snohomish County; 2012.
8. Kobler K, Limbo R, Kavanaugh K. Meaningful Moments. MCN Am J Matern Child Nurs 2007;32(5):288–97.
9. Miller J. Finding hope when a child dies: what other cultures can teach us. New York: Simon & Schuster; 1999.
10. Cacciatore J, Flint M. Mediating grief: postmortem ritualization after child death. J Loss Trauma 2012;17(2):158–72.
11. Quartier T. Deathbed rituals: roles of spiritual caregivers in Dutch hospitals. Mortality 2010;15(2):107–21.
12. Doka K. Religion and spirituality: assessment and intervention. J Soc Work End Life Palliat Care 2011;7(1):99–109.
13. Sheehan MN. Spirituality and Medicine. J Palliat Med 2003;6(3):429–31.
14. National Consensus Project for Quality Palliative Care. Clinical practice guidelines for quality palliative care. 3rd edition. Pittsbrugh (PA): National Consensus Project; 2013.
15. Ferrell BR, Borneman T. Integrating spirituality into palliative care, education, and research. Caring for the Human Spirit Magazine 2015;20–1. Sp/Su.
16. Miller J. The transforming power of spirituality. Presentation at: Conference on transformative grief. Burnsville (NC), November, 1994.
17. Lovell A. The changing identities of miscarriage and stillbirth: influences on practice and ritual. Bereavement Care 2001;20(3):37–40.
18. Lo B, Kates LW, Ruston D, et al. Responding to requests regarding prayer and religious ceremonies by patients near the end of life and their families. J Palliat Med 2003;6(3):409–15.
19. Koenig H. Religion, spirituality, and medicine: research findings and implications for clinical practice. South Med J 2004;97:1194–200.

20. Fanos JH, Little GA, Edwards WH. Candles in the snow: ritual and memory for siblings of infants who died in the intensive care nursery. J Pediatr 2009; 154(6):849–53.
21. Frøen JF, Cacciatore J, Mcclure EM, et al. Stillbirths: why they matter. Lancet 2011;377(9774):1353–66.
22. Bayley H. Finding the courage to move on. Therapy Today [serial online] 2005; 16(7):28–30. Available at: http://web.b.ebscohost.com/ehost/detail/detail? sid=9b7a3f97-b39e-43c0-824b-696c62fcb2f2%40sessionmgr104&vid=1&hid= 102&bdata=JnNpdGU9ZWhvc3QtbGl2ZQ%3d%3d#AN=19767305&db=a9h. Accessed February 29, 2016.
23. Mercurio MR. Rituals of unburdening. Hastings Cent Rep 2008;38(2):8–9.
24. McCreight BS. A grief ignored: narratives of pregnancy loss from a male perspective. Sociol Health Illn 2004;26(3):326–50.
25. Lasker JN, Toedter LJ. Satisfaction with hospital care and intervention after pregnancy loss. Death Stud 1994;18(1):41–64.
26. Benner P. Death as a human passage: compassionate care for persons dying in critical care units. Am J Crit Care 2001;10(5):355–9. Available at: http://search.proquest. com/docview/227805634/fulltext/631CFDC241E741B3PQ/1?accountid=12768. Accessed February 29, 2016.
27. Bartels JB. The pause. Crit Care Nurse 2014;34(1):74–5.
28. Quizon D. A 'pause' for reverence in the emergency room. Daily Progress 2015. Available at: http://www.dailyprogress.com/news/local/a-pause-for-reverence-in-the-emergency-room/article_46a0c244-6a11-11e5-bcf7-371adf2c4530.html. Accessed February 29, 2016.
29. O'Malley PJ, Barata IA, Snow SK. Death of a child in the emergency department. Ann Emerg Med 2014;64(1):102–5.
30. Truog RD, Christ G, Borwning DM, et al. Sudden traumatic death in children: "We did everything, but your child didn't survive." JAMA 2006;295(22):2646–54.
31. Harrison ME, Walling A. What do we know about giving bad news? A review. Clin Pediatr 2010;49(7):619–26.
32. Atwood DA. To hold her hand: Family presence during patient resuscitation. JONAS Healthc Law Ethics Regul 2006;10(1):12–6.
33. Henderson DP, Knapp JF. Report of the national consensus conference on family presence during cardiopulmonary resuscitation and procedures. Pediatr Emerg Care 2005;21(11):787–91.
34. Mangurten J, Scott SH, Guzzetta CE. Effects of family presence during resuscitation and invasive procedures in a pediatric department. J Emerg Nurs 2006; 32(3):225–33.
35. Beder J. Mourning the unfound: how we can help. J Fam Nurs 2002;83(4):400–3.
36. Boss P. Ambiguous loss. Cambridge (MA): Harvard University Press; 1999.
37. Barkas D, Voigtritter S, Shynk T. Compassion doesn't end when the heart stops: nurse's perceptions of honoring ceremony at end-of-life. Clinical Nurse Specialist 2014;28(2):E11.
38. Center for Health Equity Research and Promotion. Honoring Veterans after death: The success of the flag protocol at the White River Junction VAMC. Available at: http://www.cherp.research.va.gov/PROMISE/Honoring_Veterans_after_death_The_ success_of_the_flag_protocol_at_the_White_River_Junction_VAMC.asp. Accessed February 29, 2016.
39. Rando TA. Creating therapeutic rituals in the psychotherapy of the bereaved. Psychotherapy 1985;22(2):236.

40. Gudmundsdottir M, Chesla C. Building a new world: Habits and practices of healing following the death of a child. J Fam Nurs 2006;12(2):143–64.
41. Ruby J. Portraying the dead. Omega 1988-1989;19(1):1–20.
42. Rutenberg M. Casting the spirit: a handmade legacy. Art Ther J Am Art Ther Assoc 2008;25(3):108–14.
43. Facebook. Facebook Memorial Policies. Available at: https://www.facebook.com/help/150486848354038. Accessed February 17, 2016.
44. Nowatzki NR, Kalischuk RG. Post-death encounters: grieving, mourning, and healing. Omega 2009;59(2):91–111.
45. Berger AS. Quoth the raven: bereavement and the paranormal. Omega 1995;31(1):1–10.
46. Haraldsson E. Survey of claimed encounters with the dead. Omega 1988-1989;19(2):103–12.
47. Vickio CJ. Together in spirit: Keeping our relationships alive when loved ones die. Death Stud 1999;23(2):161–75.
48. Cohoon WD. Infant baptism: an evangelical chaplain's enlightenment. J Pastoral Care Counsel 2013;67(2):7.
49. State law officiants requirements. US Marriage Laws. Available at: http://www.usmarriagelaws.com/marriage-license/officiants-requirements.shtml. Accessed February 23, 2016.
50. Alaska Nurses Association. 'I Do' at the Bedside. Alaska Nurse 2013;63(4):5. Available at: http://ezproxy.library.nyu.edu:2138/ehost/pdfviewer/pdfviewer?sid=7a652b05-c4b4-4997-8615-65e8b59278df%40sessionmgr4001&vid=1&hid=4207. Accessed February 29, 2016.
51. Hatchett MJ. Commentary on the American prayer book. New York: The Seabury Press; 1980.
52. Potvin N. The role of music therapy and ritual drama in transformation during imminent death. Music Ther Perspect 2015;33(1):53–62.
53. Moodley R, Costa I. Teddy bears, flowers and crucifixes: collective responses to trauma. Int J Health Promot Educ 2006;44(1):38–42.
54. Bondi SA. The birthday party. JAMA Pediatr 2013;167(1):7.
55. Bourgeois S, Johnson A. Preparing for dying: meaningful practices in palliative care. Omega 2004;49(2):99–107.
56. Heyse-Moore L. On spiritual pain in the dying. Mortality 1996;1(3):297–315, 19p.
57. Fristad MA, Cerel J, Goldman M, et al. The role of ritual in children's bereavement. Omega 2000-2001;42(4):321–39.
58. Delbene R. Into the light: a simple way to pray with the sick and dying. Nashville (TN): The Upper Room; 1988.
59. Blum CA. 'Til death do us part?' the nurse's role in the care of the dead. Geriatr Nurs 2006;27(1):58–63.
60. Kobler K. Leaning in and holding on: team support with unexpected death. MCN Am J Matern Child Nurs 2014;39(3):148–54.
61. Papadatou D. In the face of death: professionals who are for the dying and the bereaved. New York: Springer Publishing Company; 2009.

APPENDIX 1: GIVING THANKS FOR THE UNEXPECTED LOSS OF A LIFE

(Opening salutation—[Almighty God, Creator God, Merciful Father, Loving Source of Being, G_d of grace and glory]), we gather to give thanks for [name *or* this child]. We thank you for giving *him* to us, *his* family and friends, to know and to love. Console *us/those* who care for [name] and who now mourn. Give us the courage and strength to see in death ever new possibilities in life so that we may continue forward. We give thanks for those who have been called to the arts of healing and the prevention of pain and disease. Strengthen us so that our work/ministries of health to the community may continue. In your holy name, we pray. Amen.

A closing ritual at the bedside of the deceased

I thank everyone here for your compassionate care and your efforts to do everything possible for (name of patient). Let us take a moment in silence to acknowledge our sorrow at (his/her) death. …Let us rededicate ourselves to the honor and the wonder of the work that we do.

From O'Malley PJ, Barata IA, Snow SK. Death of a child in the emergency department. Ann Emerg Med 2014;64(1):102–05.

APPENDIX 2: IN THE CASE OF THE NEED FOR EMERGENCY BAPTISM
Supplies needed

A bowl, water, towel (bed pads may be used if significant amounts of water are to be poured over the candidate for baptism), baptismal certificate (can be kept on hand in unit/location).

A formula for emergency baptism

1. Pour water into bowl; bless the water with these or similar words: "We thank you, Almighty God, for the gift of water. Water leads us through death and resurrection and from this life into the eternal. Bless this water we pray you by the power of your Holy Spirit."
2. Presentation and naming [by parents/sponsors]: "I/We present [name] for the rite of baptism."
3. Prayer (optional): "May [name] be delivered from all sin and all evil and opened to grace and truth, filled with God's life-giving Spirit, and brought to the fullness of God's eternal life and peace."
4. Rite of baptism: "*I baptize you in the Name of the Father* [sprinkling/pouring water over the candidate for baptism] *and of the Son, and of the Holy Spirit. Amen.*"
5. Closing prayer: "Heavenly Father we thank you that by water and the Holy Spirit you have bestowed on this your servant the forgiveness of sin and have raised him/her to new life of grace. [name], you have been marked as Christ's own forever." Amen.

Adapted from Church Publishing. The book of common prayer and administration of the sacraments and other rites and ceremonies of the church. New York: Oxford University Press; 1979.

Seeing the Light

End-of-Life Experiences—Visions, Energy Surges, and Other Death Bed Phenomena

Dorothy Wholihan, DNP, AGPCNP-BC, GNP-BC, ACHPN

KEYWORDS

- Death bed phenomenon • Visions • Premortem surge • End-of-life dreams
- Hallucinations

KEY POINTS

- Death bed phenomena are common within the last days and weeks of life and can include visions, dreams, hallucinations, and premortem energy surges.
- These end-of-life experiences have been underrecognized and unappreciated by health care providers, often discounted as the results of medical delirium.
- General consensus among those describing these death bed occurrences is that they are a source of consolation to dying patients and families.
- Qualitative studies show that patients and families are often more likely to talk about these experiences to nurses than to other health care providers.
- Nursing interventions to normalize and validate these phenomena and open channels of communication can impact care during this period and facilitate a more peaceful passing.

Mr. B was a 77-year-old widower with advanced lung cancer who was admitted to our hospice unit. Frequently, on morning rounds he spoke about seeing his deceased wife during the night. She never spoke to him, but he found her presence very soothing. One day he described how she came and helped him into the wheelchair and took him to the hospital chapel, where his breathing difficulties resolved, and his chronic anxiety lessened.

—Hospice nurse

I could tell my mother was close to death; she was much less responsive, her breathing was becoming more difficult, and she only took occasional sips of water. At a few points during those last few days, she would arouse herself and speak a few words, talking to my father and my sister, although he had been dead for 5 years and my sister was out of the country. I rubbed her shoulder and told

Disclosure Statement: The authors have nothing to disclose.
NYU College of Nursing, 433 First Avenue, New York, NY 10011, USA
E-mail address: dw57@nyu.edu

her I was there with her. She smiled and said, "Great! We are having a wonderful time!

—Daughter of patient who died in a nursing home.

INTRODUCTION AND HISTORY

End-of-life experiences have been defined through various terms: death bed phenomenon, death bed visions, death bed dreams, near-death experiences, and nearing death awareness.[1] These end-of-life visions and dreams have been documented throughout history and across cultures.[2,3] End-of-life experiences are found in biographies and literature of all ages, from ancient Egyptian coffin design to the sightings of medieval Christian mystics and saints.[4] Paintings depict Saint Francis of Assisi on his death bed, reaching out to monks who welcome him to heaven.[5] The 14th century English mystic Julian of Norwich was struck with a life-threatening illness during a time of plague and experienced 16 religious vision preparing her for death and reassuring her—"all shall be well."[6] In *The Death of Ivan Ilyich*, Tolstoy describes Ivan's deathbed experience, writing, "In place of death, there was light. 'So that's what it is!' he suddenly exclaimed aloud, 'What joy!'"[7(pp58)] More recently, Elizabeth Kubler-Ross, in her groundbreaking work, *On Death and Dying*, discovered numerous examples of death bed phenomenon in her pioneering interviews of terminally ill patients.[8]

The general consensus among those describing these death bed experiences is that they are a source of consolation to dying patients and their families,[9] yet until recently, they have been largely discounted by the health care establishment. This article aims to summarize past research into end-of-life experiences—visions, dreams, hallucinations, and premortem energy surges—with the goal of increasing the clinical understanding and implications for the bedside clinician.

BARRIERS TO RECOGNITION OF THE CLINICAL SIGNIFICANCE OF END-OF-LIFE EXPERIENCES

Historically, the phenomena of dreams, visions, and energy surges have not been analyzed fully or integrated into the care of patients at the end of life. These end-of-life experiences have been frequently dismissed as the physiologic effects of medications, hypoxia, infection, metabolic disturbances, or other causes of delirium.[3] When an end-of-life experience is clearly manifested, the experience is often unreported, ignored by staff or family, or the patient medicated with antipsychotic or tranquilizing medications. Little attempt has been made to deeply assess the occurrence or to analyze the clinical significance.

The dearth of information about this phenomenon has resulted from a variety of barriers, including patient and family reluctance to report these events and staff failure to engage in assessment or discussion, often stemming fear of ridicule on the parts of all involved.

Furthermore, in a culturally diverse patient population, patients and families may not have adequate language skills to clearly communicate these vague perceptions. One hospice staff member describes why death bed phenomena are so difficult to explain within a medical model: "we just don't have the language to describe it, and that's the reason we don't investigate it."[10(pp21)] **Table 1** lists the common barriers to recognition of the clinical significance of end-of-life experiences.

REVIEW OF THE LITERATURE

A literature search was conducted from 2000 on to evaluate the status of the current literature exploring death bed phenomena and end-of-life experiences. Because there

Table 1	
Barriers to recognition of clinical significance of death bed phenomena	
Patient and Family Barriers	**Clinician Barriers**
Embarrassment/fear of ridicule	Embarrassment/fear of ridicule
Fear of distressing relatives	Doubts about medical legitimacy; professional skepticism
Weakness and debility of patients	Lack of time for deep discussions
Fear of appearing crazy	Inability to recognize significance of experience
Inadequacy of language to describe experience	Lack of education/training about spiritual care at end of life
Lack of privacy in institutional settings	Personal discomfort with communicating about death
Not routinely asked about end-of-life experiences	—

Adapted from Refs.[3,5,10].

are no well-defined terms for these phenomena, an iterative and extensive keyword search was initially carried out for several computerized databases. This search helped to accurately determine which search terms best captured the desired subject. In all, 24 terms were used. The most productive search terms included death bed communication, death bed dream, death bed vision, death bed escort, meaning-centered dream, predeath vision, and death-related sensory experience.

In general, there exists a dearth of research about the phenomenon of end-of-life experiences. Most of the findings are presented as literary work, often geared toward the lay public, with anecdotal reports of unusual phenomenon witnessed by health care staff and family.[11,12] *Final Gifts*, a book describing the personal experiences of 2 hospice nurses, offers their personal interpretation of "Nearing Death Awareness" along with advice about increasing attentiveness to this phenomenon, with the aim of a more meaningful experience for family. Popular with a lay audience and a best-seller upon its release, *Final Gifts* is a collection of clinical anecdotes, along with personal interpretation.[13]

There has been a scarcity of studies asking patients directly for first-hand accounts of their experiences, and fewer still demonstrate any scholarly rigor. However, interest in this topic is broad ranged and stems from a wide array of fields, including palliative medicine, nursing,[9,10,14] psychiatry,[4,5,15] and religious studies.[16]

INCIDENCE

Reports of the prevalence of death bed phenomena in dying patients vary depending on who is surveyed: health care staff or patients and family directly. Muthumana[2] summarizes the difficulties in estimating prevalence of death bed phenomena encountered in past research. Studies have been mostly retrospective, sometimes involving long-term recollection. They are often based reports of professionals, rather than the patients themselves or family who are more consistently present, and results are often obtained from opportunistic, rather than systematic representative sampling. In an effort to define the prevalence of death bed visions, the researcher interviewed caregivers in a community hospice in India within 2 weeks of their family member's death. This study found 40 of 104 families (38%) reported "unusual experiences or behaviors" involving interaction with deceased relatives. Although the sample size was not large (n = 40), statistical analysis of demographics was performed. No difference in occurrence of visions was found in terms of age, gender, earlier occupation, place of death, or use of opioid medication. Religion did affect the experience, with more Hindus than Muslims reporting visions. Of the 40 death bed phenomena reported, 30 included visions of deceased family and friends, 6 were clear premonitions of imminent death, and 4 were unclear confusional states felt to be owing to delirium and involving dark shadows and insects.

Fountain[17] interviewed patients and families to determine the prevalence and describe the experience of hallucinations in 100 hospice patients. She found that 47% of patients reported visual hallucinations in the month before the interview, one-half of which occurred frequently, at least several times per week. Evaluating this phenomenon from a medical framework, the researcher reported clear differences in the types of visions. Most common (43%) were hallucinations involving familiar people standing at the bedside, usually experienced in relation to falling asleep or waking, and reported as nonfrightening. Alternatively, hallucinations were also reported during recovery from periods of delirium, where the visions were more unpleasant, continuous, and involved animals or objects. Unfortunately, this study did not report on any correlation between risk factors and type of hallucination (ie, comforting or distressing). So, although general risk factors were discovered in this study, one cannot detail which factors lead to positive or negative experiences. Further research is needed to explore the significance of risk factors in connection to various experiences.

Higher level prospective research into the phenomenon is lacking, but several qualitative studies do exist. Fenwick and Brayne[4] in the United Kingdom are among those conducting the most work in the area of what they term as "end-of-life experiences."[5,10,18] From an initial pilot study interviewing hospice workers, Brayne, Farnham, and Fenwick[10] learned that these experiences occur relatively frequently and that patients and family tend to talk about them to nurses rather than doctors. The researchers later completed 3 further full-scale qualitative studies of care providers, including both retrospective and prospective studies using interview, questionnaire and diary records of interdisciplinary hospice staff.

In 2010, Fenwick, Lovelace, and Brayne[4] studied the experiences and attitudes of 38 interdisciplinary providers in hospices and nursing homes, both retrospectively and prospectively, and found that 62% of these caregivers reported that dying patients or their relatives reported death bed visions to them. Eighty-nine percent of respondents believed that these visions were a profound spiritual experience for patients and families, with fewer believing they resulted from medication or fever (35%), or a chemical change in the brain (31%).

In 2007, an article was written in the British newspaper *The Daily Mail*[19] reporting on the ongoing work of Fenwick and colleagues as described here. As a result of this publicity, the researchers received more than 700 letters and emails from bereaved friends, relatives, and caregivers in response to the article. This response surely demonstrates that although the medical establishment has traditionally responded to these reports with skepticism, the lay public views them as true phenomenon. The researchers analyzed the content of a sampling of these emails, 85% of which were first-hand accounts of witnesses. Analysis of these emails revealed similar themes to their previously published work: that the visions were primarily of family (most commonly siblings, then parents), that they occurred at various times, but more often within 12 to 24 hours before death, and that the overwhelming majority of witnessed felt the dying patient was happy to see the apparitions. Both family members and patients were reassured and comforted by the experience.[18]

Kerr and colleagues[3] conducted a prospective longitudinal mixed methods study using semistructured interviews of hospice in-patients from admission to death. Patients were daily asked a 7-item survey and open-ended questions to obtain quantitative and descriptive data. In this study, 59 patients reported a total of 276 instances of dreams and visions, 45% occurring during sleep, portraying realistic visions of deceased and living friends, family, pets, or a combination thereof. Eighty-eight percent of the sample interviewed experienced at least 1 end-of-life experience, a 2-fold increase from past studies that only interviewed family and staff. Almost 20% of patients experienced multiple episodes in a given day. Researchers found a significant correlation between seeing deceased or mixed living/deceased loved ones and feelings of solace and comfort. Most patients reported that deceased loved ones offered guidance and reassurance, although not always verbal. The frequency of these experiences increased significantly as death approached. Interestingly, 59% of patients described visions that included themes of preparing to go someplace (eg, involving walking somewhere, driving in cars), and only a few included religious content or symbols.

The phenomenon of premortem surge (a burst of energy right before death) has not been studied extensively, although anecdotal accounts have been published.[11,13,15] In preparation for their study, Schreiber and Bennett[20] failed to identify any study of this particular death bed phenomenon. They went on to conduct a Delphi study to systematically collect observations and perceptions of the experience from a panel of certified and advanced certified hospice and palliative nurses. Three rounds of Delphi surveys were completed, involving 64 expert panelists. These surveys were used to generate a consensus of identified characteristics and nursing implications.

The research into death bed phenomenon, like so much work in palliative care, involves small sample sizes of fragile and vulnerable people. Yet, there exist many consistencies among these studies, including the prevalence of visions of known deceased loved ones and acquaintances and the sense of comfort and peace obtained from these visions. Additionally, the work of several researchers demonstrates that these death-related sensory experiences cross cultures and religions.[2,21] In addition, Ethier[14] studied the phenomena in a pediatric oncology population and found that children also draw comfort from death bed visions, often with a preponderance of angelic figures. In light of these common findings in varying populations, it behooves the nurse to understand the implications of the phenomenon and explore how to integrate these experiences into care so as to facilitate peaceful death.

DEFINING DEATH BED PHENOMENA: VISIONS

Hospice nurses Callanan and Kelley defined the term "Nearing Death Awareness" in their book, *Final Gifts*, which consists of anecdotes from their years of practice and is written for the general public.[13] In this book, they categorize death bed visions into 2 distinct forms. The most common visions are of spirits (usually deceased friends and relatives) who greet and encourage the dying: "these spirits may visit for minutes or even hours; they are not seen by those at the bedside of the dying person, but it is often obvious that the dying person is communicating with an unseen presence."[13(pp38)] These visions are usually personal in their cultural, religious, and historical context. Appropriate religious symbols and historical personalities are linked with the individuals' backgrounds. Staff interviewed often considered the prognostic implications of death bed visions and the limited evidence does suggest that these phenomena occur more frequently as death approaches.[10,18]

The second type is a vision concerning transitioning to the place where the dying believe they are headed. These visions are usually glowing and brief: the so-called light at the end of the tunnel. Included also in this category are visions involving symbols of transportation, such as trains[10] or airplanes.[22] Animals at times are present in these visions, appearing around the time of death. Fenwick, Lovelace, and Brayne describe a woman's vision of a small bird, "She asked me to open the window and I did, and she said: 'That bird will take my soul,'"[18(pp176)]

Several authors note the difference between death bed phenomenon and the sensations encountered during a near death experience.[13,16] Near death experiences are felt by those who have suffered a potentially fatal event, but who do not die. Frequently, the visions seen are similar in their composition, as comforting, reassuring symbols and communications. Near death experiences inform current understanding of death bed phenomena, but the experiences are inherently different for dying patients: "These are people on a journey towards death, not people who just missed it."[23]

DEFINING DEATH BED PHENOMENA: ENERGY SURGES IN THE LAST HOURS OF LIFE

Caregivers and family also describe episodes of previously confused or semiconscious patients having a brief moment of lucidity enabling them to say their farewells.[5] This phenomenon has been coined "premortem surge" and has been reported to occur as a sudden, unexpected, inexplicable period of increased energy and enhanced mental clarity that can occur hours to days before death, varying in intensity and duration.[20] Some authors use the term "terminal lucidity" to describe this phenomenon.[15,18] Emanuel and colleagues[11(pp3)] described the event as a "burst of energy or golden glow" that indicated impending death. The expert consensus reported by Schreiber and Bennett in their Delphi study indicated that premortem surge is an observable phenomenon that occurs frequently, but unpredictably. It is described as a 1-time event appearing up to 48 hours before death, and lasting from 6 to 24 hours. During the experience, a previously moribund patient awakes and exhibits improved mentation, an ability to communicate, and an interest in eating, without distress or agitation. Consensus also indicates that family often observe this phenomenon and are mostly comforted by the pleasant experience, which at times is considered a gift. However, families at times may be confused by the surge and can experience resulting feelings of alarm. Uncertainty, false hope, and regret about previous decisions about treatment can occur if the experience is not put into proper perspective and its temporary presence appreciated.[20]

DEATH BED PHENOMENA: MYSTICAL EXPERIENCES OR MEDICAL DELIRIUM?

Thanatological scholars argue for the reality of these visions: that these "spirits" are real phenomenon, rather than the results of medical decline or hallucinations; hallucinations are described as the seeing or hearing of things that are not real.[16] Theologians such as Betty[16] contend that such visions may in fact be real, given the impressive sense of reality felt, and the sheer numbers reported (even by atheists who do not believe in life after death). Alternatively, delirious hallucinations are described by some as more hazy and distorted, and often produce anxiety or distress.[9] In their hospice study, Brayne and colleagues[10] interviewed interdisciplinary staff who clearly differentiated between the experiences of death bed visions and delirium-induced hallucinations. They reported that drug-induced hallucinations were more likely to be annoying or frightening images of animals, unfamiliar children, insects, or malevolent figures like devils and dragons, some obviously derived from distortions of items in the immediate environment. They report that patients who see medical hallucinations frequently acknowledge seeing things that are not real, whereas death bed visions are connected vividly to realities of their life and frequently hold deeper meaning to them. Obviously, the paranormal versus medical causes of these phenomena will not be easily resolved. The ultimate etiology of these phenomena is only relevant in shaping clinical response to them.

IMPLICATIONS FOR PRACTICE
Clinical Assessment of Death Bed Phenomena

In her study of hospice patients experiencing hallucinations, Fountain[17] analyzed risk factors associated with hallucinations, finding a trend (although not statistically significant) toward increased hallucinations in patients receiving opioids or other medications known to have the potential for neurologic side effects. Other risk factors included presence of brain tumors, renal failure, or underlying psychiatric disorders. Interestingly, no correlation was found between experience of hallucination and cognitive impairment as measured by the Mini-Mental Status Examination. Overall, hallucinating patients had 5.19 risk factors and at least 3 high-risk medications. There was not a single patient whose hallucinations could be attributed solely to opioids. This can reassure clinicians about the need to continue adequate analgesic in the last hours of life.

Death bed phenomena should be assessed and addresses according to the basic principles of symptom management. First, the goals of care must be clarified or confirmed. If the goal is comfort only, the experience must be evaluated within this framework. A vision that is comforting in itself needs no intervention. If distress or unrest results from the experience, a workup and determination of the potential cause may be indicated, and medications may be administered to address patient suffering caused by the experience. In addition, any associated symptoms or behaviors must be assessed. Does the phenomenon lead to increased agitation or dyspnea? Does the patient try to reach out or get out of bed to go to the vision? Does the premortem surge lead to increased fall risk? Assessment parameters are listed in **Box 1**.

Open Communication

Nurses caring for dying patients find the end-of-life experiences of their patients such as death bed visions "neither rare or surprising."[4] Qualitative studies show that patients and families are often more likely to talk about these experiences to nurses, rather than to doctors.[10] Yet educational preparation about care in the last hours of life is lacking, and nurses often lack the time and training to be able to respond to such phenomena in ways that achieve maximal therapeutic effect. Being able to recognize and respond to death bed phenomenon can greatly influence the nurse's impact on care during this crucial period. The willingness to actively assess these experiences, overcome the traditional medically oriented view, and embrace the spiritual side of end-of-life care is integral to being able to comfortably facilitate these discussions. As one interviewee remarked, "if it doesn't fit my previous preconceived ideas, I try to still hear it, and see if I can incorporate it somehow in how I communicate with them."[10(pp22)]

CARE OF FAMILY AND LOVED ONES

Betty[16] describes how family can view visions as a gift for their own future. Although not direct participants, they witness the comfort attained by the patient and the messages conveyed by the visions experienced by the dying patient. This can positively affect their own perceptions of death and dying. Callanan and Kelley[13(pp102)] quote

---

Box 1
Assessment of death bed phenomenon

1. Patient and family reports of phenomenon (direct questioning of patients is most effective assessment)
   - Address in calm, matter-of-fact manner:
     - "How have you been sleeping?"
     - "Can you recall any dreams while you were sleeping or just resting?"
     - "Have you encountered anything out of the ordinary lately?"
   - Are visions disorganized or is there meaning?
   - Are visions familiar to the patient (ie, deceased friends or relatives)?
   - Are visions of animals, insects, or frightening images?
   - Does this dream/vision bring comfort or distress?

2. Presence of risk factors that may predispose patient to distressing hallucinations
   - Past diagnosis of PTSD or history of trauma (which might predispose patient to undiagnosed PTSD).
   - Polypharmacy with medications affecting the CNS (ie, high-dose steroids, opioid toxicity).
   - Poorly managed physical symptoms (ie, dyspnea, pain, urinary retention, constipation/impaction).
   - Disease states predisposing to delirium (ie, brain metastasis, hepatic failure, hypercalcemia).

3. Assess risk of complications associated with witnessing visions (ie, increased movements leading to pain or fall risk).

4. Assess and address patient's emotional response or distress resulting from visions

5. Assess and address emotional response of witnesses (family, significant others, roommates, care providers).

Abbreviations: CNS, central nervous system; PTSD, posttraumatic stress disorder.
  Data from Refs.[3,9,20,23]

---

one family member: "because Bobby's death was so peaceful. I'll never be as scared of death ... he gave me a little preview of what lay beyond it for him, and I hope, for me."

Specific attention must be directed toward the family and loved ones who witness the phenomenon of premortem surge at the end of life. This unexpected improvement in a patient's level of energy and alertness can provide the opportunity for last good-byes and meaningful closure.[24] The opportunity to complete unfinished tasks and final leave taking can result in family interpretation of the event as a "last gift to them and they did not question the logic of it."[20(pp433)] However, some families develop false hope of unexpected recovery and develop last minute doubts about previously established goals of care. Informed nurses can be on the lookout for symptoms of premortem surge and educate families for them to develop realistic expectations and make effective use of the short-lived time together. Interventions for family care witnessing death bed phenomena are listed in **Box 2**.

PATIENTS

Fountain[17(pp24)] writes, "Most patients, even very ill ones, readily talked about their visual hallucinations when asked about them and welcomed the opportunity to do so. Many were comforted by the reassurance that hallucinations are common experiences, and that they were not going mad." Open discussions of the phenomena and educating patients that these are common occurrences can help to normalize the experience and reassure patients and family.

Box 2
Supporting families who witness death bed phenomena

1. Maintain open channels of communication by use of open ended questions and empathic listening skills.

2. Maintain an accepting attitude and normalize the experience when assessing and discussing experiences:
   - "We see many patients who experience dreams and visions at this time—have you noticed this about your loved one?"
   - "It is common for patient to talk to people who have died. Let's see what we can learn by listening."

3. Provide written information about the last weeks, days, and hours of life

4. *Use validating language*: "I can see this is perplexing to you."

5. Assist family to find comforting meaning in visions, if possible.

6. If visions are distressing, *treat suffering*
   - Ask family about patient's past traumatic events.
   - Consult with interprofessional team to evaluate if anxiolytic or antipsychotic medications and/or intensive spiritual or psychotherapeutic interventions are indicated.

7. Facilitate communication about the experience between patient and family, if desired and appropriate.

8. Incorporate early and active collaboration with interprofessionals and available spiritual care providers, encouraging staff analysis of experience.

9. Referral to community resources such as community spiritual care providers, local bereavement groups or online supports (ie, Griefnet.org, cancercare.org).

Data from Mazzarino-Willet A. Deathbed phenomenon: its role in peaceful death and terminal restlessness. Am J Hosp Palliat Care 2010;27:127–33; and Hoffman J. A new vision for dreams of the dying. New York Times. 2016. Available at: http://www.nytimes.com/2016/02/02/health/dreams-dying-deathbed-interpretation-delirium.html; http://www.nytimes.com/2016/02/02/health/dreams-dying-deathbed-%09interpretation-delirium.html?mwrsm=Email. Accessed February 2, 2016.

Fenwick and Brayne[18] highlight the importance of recognizing that most death bed visions involve people to whom the dying person felt a close emotional affinity, suggesting that the human need for close connections and loving acceptance is as strong at death as it is earlier in life. This interpretation mandates closer human contact between nurses and patients at this crucial time of passing.

The common vision of previously deceased loved ones is an especially important aspect for nurses to consider. Nurses can recognize and acknowledge these connections, so as to inspire hope in patients and families, and recognize that these deeply spiritual connections between loved ones may provide a link between this world and the next. These appearances can have an intense and lasting effect by bringing hope to patients and families: hope of an onward journey, rather than absolute finality.[18] Such exchanges provide occasions for empathy and support, as well as a time for validation and normalization. Both dying patients and families benefit from understanding that death bed experiences are usual in circumstances of dying and that our understanding of these encounters in in its infancy.[2]

Even if nurses themselves do not hold strong beliefs in an afterlife, they can recognize and accept the meanings held by their patients and families. Nursing assessment and interventions to validate these phenomena can help facilitate a more peaceful passing. More than any other member of the health care team, nurses are in the unique position to be an active and connected presence during this transition, especially for patients without supports at the bedside.

NEED FOR EDUCATION

Despite increasing recognition and research documenting the occurrences of this phenomenon, the topic is not covered routinely in traditional health professional curricula. In Fenwick, Lovelace, and Brayne's survey of health care providers, only 17% reported receiving any training about end-of-life experiences.[4] Consequently, many medical and nursing providers felt ill-equipped to address these spiritual death bed experiences, a response that correlates with the reports of nurses in general about feelings of inadequacy in the provision of spiritual care.[25]

As a result of limited education and nurses' low self-efficacy with regard to spiritual care, many death bed experiences that are intensely meaningful are often dismissed as insignificant. They are considered within the medical model and believed to be either confusional or drug induced and have no intrinsic value.[4] However, as Betty[15(pp48)] admonishes: "If we don't make the mistake of assuming they are 'confused', we are likely to feel some of the excitement they convey.... for we are witnessing the momentary merging of two worlds." Nurse Mazzarino-Willet[9(pp132)] opines, "All health care clinicians need to become masters in the art of active listening." Increased education in end-of-life care, with emphasis on spirituality, can raise awareness and acceptance of the occurrence of death bed phenomena, allowing nurses to open the door for communication with patients and families.

SUMMARY

Spiritual care is an integral part of multidimensional palliative care, and is one of the major domains of care identified in well-established definitions and guidelines.[26–28] Death bed visions and other phenomena can be deeply spiritual experiences for patients, family, and staff, yet have historically been underrecognized and unappreciated by health care providers. The last hours of life are a sacred time, and as holistic, multidimensional practitioners, nurses should remain open to experiences not easily explained within our traditional medical model. As the most consistent caregivers, around the clock and at the bedside, nurses are charged with the responsibility to assess, recognize, and validate such extraordinary experiences, to assist patients in finding meaning, comfort, and a dignified and peaceful end of life.

ACKNOWLEDGMENTS

The author acknowledges the invaluable contribution of S. Abrames for his extensive research and review of the current evidence included in this paper.

REFERENCES

1. Corless IB. Transitions: exploring the frontier. Omega 2014;70:57–65.
2. Muthumana SP, Kumar M, Kellehear A, et al. Deathbed visions from India: a study of family observations in northern Kerala. Omega 2014;32:97–109.
3. Kerr CW, Donnelly JP, Wright ST, et al. End-of-life dreams and visions: a longitudinal study of hospice patients' experiences. J Palliat Med 2014;17:296–303.
4. Fenwick P, Brayne S. End-of-life experiences: reaching out for compassion, communication, and connection – meaning of deathbed visions and coincidences. Am J Hosp Palliat Care 2011;28:7–15.

5. Fenwick P, Lovelace H, Brayne S. End of life experiences and their implications for palliative care. Int J Environ Stud 2007;64:315–23.
6. Underhill E. Julian of Norwich. In: The essentials of mysticism. 1920. Available at: www.ccel.org/search/fulltext/julian%20of%20norwich%20. Accessed January 18, 2015.
7. Tolstoy LV. The death of Ivan Ilyich. Hazelton (PA): Penn State University Electronics Classics Series Publications; 1886. Available at: http://opie.wvnet.edu/~jelkins/lawyerslit/stories/death-of-ivan-ilych.pdf. Accessed January 18, 2016.
8. Kubler-Ross E. On death and dying. New York: Scribner Publishers; 1969.
9. Mazzarino-Willet A. Deathbed phenomenon: its role in peaceful death and terminal restlessness. Am J Hosp Palliat Care 2010;27:127–33.
10. Brayne S, Farnham C, Fenwick P. Deathbed phenomena and their effect on a palliative care team: A Pilot Study. Am J Hosp Palliat Care 2006;23:17–24.
11. Emanuel, L, Ferris, F, von Gunten, C, et al. The last hours of living: practical advice for clinicians. Medscape Nursing Website. 2010. Available at: www.medscape.org/viewarticle/716874. Accessed February 1, 2016.
12. Lerma J. Into the light. Pompton Plains (NJ): New Page Books; 2007.
13. Callanan M, Kelley P. Final gifts. New York: Bantam Publishing; 1992.
14. Ethier AM. Death-related sensory experiences. J Pediatr Oncol Nurs 2005;22:104–11.
15. Nahm M, Greyson B, Kelly EW, et al. Terminal lucidity: a review and a case collection. Arch Gerontol Geriatr 2012;55:138–42.
16. Betty LS. Are they hallucinations or are they real? The spirituality of deathbed and near-death visions. Omega 2006;53:37–49.
17. Fountain A. Visual hallucinations: a prevalence study among hospice inpatients. Palliat Med 2001;15:19–25.
18. Fenwick P, Lovelace H, Brayne S. Comfort for the dying: five year retrospective and one year prospective studies of end of life experiences. Arch Gerontol Geriatr 2010;51:173–9.
19. Penman D. The angels of death. Daily Mail 2007. Available at: www.dailymail.co.uk/news/article-436808/The-Angels-Death.html. Accessed January 16, 2015.
20. Schreiber TP, Bennett MJ. Identification and validation of premortem surge. J Hosp Palliat Nurs 2014;16:40–437.
21. Kellehear A, Pogonet V, Mindruta-Stratan R, et al. Deathbed visions from the Republic of Moldova: a content analysis of family observations. Omega 2011–2012;64:303–17.
22. Nosek CL, Kerr CW, Woodworth J, et al. End-of-life dreams and visions: a qualitative perspective from hospice patients. Am J Hosp Palliat Care 2014;32:269–74.
23. Hoffman J. A new vision for dreams of the dying. New York Times 2016. Available at: www.nytimes.com/2016/02/02/health/dreams-dying-deathbed-interpretation-delirium.html?mwrsm=Email http://www.nytimes.com/2016/02/02/health/dreams-dying-deathbed-%09interpretation-delirium.html?mwrsm=Email. Accessed February 2, 2016.
24. Moneymaker K. Understanding the dying process: transitions during the final days to hours. J Palliat Med 2005;22:1079–86.
25. Molzahn AE, Shields L. Why is it so hard to talk about spirituality? Can Nurs 2008;104:25–9.
26. Pulchalski C, Ferrel BR, Virani R. Improving the quality of spiritual care as a dimension of palliative care: the report of the Consensus Conference. J Palliat Med 2009;12:885–904.

27. National Comprehensive Cancer Network (NCCN). NCCN clinical practice guidelines in oncology. 2016. Available at: www.nccn.org/professionals/physician_gls/pdf/palliative.pdf. Accessed January 31, 2016.

28. Sepulveda C, Marlin A, Yoshida T, et al. Palliative care: the World Health Organization's global perspective. J Pain Symptom Manage 2002;24:91–6.

Providing Palliative Care to LGBTQ Patients

Nina Barrett, NP, AGPCNP-BC, ACHPN[a],*,
Dorothy Wholihan, DNP, AGPCNP-BC, GNP-BC, ACHPN[b]

KEYWORDS

- LGBTQ • End-of-life • Palliative care

KEY POINTS

- LGBTQ patients have unique health issues, including higher predisposition to certain chronic illnesses and stress-sensitive mental health issues.
- The physical and mental health disparities that exist today are rooted in and reflective of a long history of discrimination and bias against LGBTQ people, at a societal level and within the health care system.
- Fear of substandard treatment results in a hesitation among LGBTQ people to reveal their sexual orientation or gender identity to health care providers. This lack of disclosure can lead to distress or compromised care.
- Effectively serving LGBTQ patients requires clinicians to understand the cultural context of their patients' lives, and modify practice policies and environments to be welcoming and inclusive.
- Nurses can provide compassionate and professional care to LGBTQ people by taking comprehensive and nonjudgmental histories, educating themselves about unique health issues, and reflecting and correcting personal attitudes that might inhibit optimal care.

Who will be there for us, who will help care for us without judgment?
—66-year-old lesbian[1]

One of the basic tenets of palliative care is the recognition that this type of care must be provided in a culturally competent manner, and that diverse populations have unique needs. All nurses should be familiar with and well equipped to address the distinct challenges that may arise when caring for lesbian, gay, bisexual, transgender, and queer-identified (LGBTQ) patients.

Estimates vary, but data gleaned from the latest United States census indicate that approximately 2% of adults age 50 and older, or about 2 million people, self-identify as

Disclosure Statement: The authors have nothing to disclose.
[a] New York Presbyterian-Columbia University Medical Center, 601 West 168th Street, 3rd Floor, #38, New York, NY 10032, USA; [b] Palliative Care Specialty Program, NYU College of Nursing, 433 First Avenue, New York, NY 10010, USA
* Corresponding author.
E-mail address: nrb2130@cumc.columbia.edu

Nurs Clin N Am 51 (2016) 501–511
http://dx.doi.org/10.1016/j.cnur.2016.05.001
0029-6465/16/$ – see front matter © 2016 Elsevier Inc. All rights reserved.

lesbian, gay, or bisexual. The population of lesbian, gay, bisexual, and transgender older adults is expected to double between 2000 and 2030, with estimates ranging from 2 to 6 million adults 65 years or older by the year 2030.[1]

UNIQUE HEALTH ISSUES

In decades past, most palliative care provided to the LGBTQ population was primarily focused on caring for patients with Human Immunodeficiency Virus (HIV)/AIDS. Although this disease continues to affect the LGBTQ population disproportionately (particularly men who have sex with men and male-to-female transgendered persons), important medical advances have made it so that HIV is now largely managed as a chronic illness.[2] In addition to HIV/AIDS, certain portions of the LGBTQ population are predisposed to other chronic, life-limiting illnesses. For example, higher rates of smoking among gay men and lesbians has correlated with increased rates of lung and bladder cancers, and lesbians are more likely to get endometrial and breast cancer than straight women.[3] The National LGBT Health and Aging Center found that LGBTQ elders have higher rates of disability than their heterosexual peers.[1]

In addition to increased rates of certain physical maladies, LGBTQ individuals are also at greater risk of suffering from a myriad of stress-sensitive mental health issues, including anxiety, depression, posttraumatic stress disorder, and suicidality.[4] There is an increased risk for abuse of alcohol and illicit drugs in this population, and the physical and mental disorders that tend to stem from this abuse.[5] Researchers postulate that negative social attitudes, widespread discrimination and stigma, higher rates of sexual assault,[6] and physical and psychological victimization contribute to these disturbing findings.[4,7] **Box 1** summarizes statistics about the unique health issues facing LGBTQ patients.

Box 1
Unique health issues facing LBGTQ patients

LGBTQ STATISTICS

- 82% have been victimized at least once in their lives
- 68% experienced verbal harassment
- 43% were threatened with violence
- 41% have a disability
- 30% do not have a will
- 36% have not appointed a health care proxy

ACCESS TO CARE STATISTICS

- 21% do not disclose their sexual orientation or gender identity to their physician
- 15% fear accessing health care outside the LGBTQ community
- 13% have been denied health care or have been provided with inferior health care
- 22% of transgender older adults need to see a doctor but cannot afford it

Data from Fredriksen-Goldsen KI, Kim HJ, Emlet CA, et al. The aging in health report: disparities and resilience among lesbian, gay, bisexual, and transgender older adults. Institute for Multigenerational Health. 2011. Available at: http://www.agingcenter.org/resources/pdfs/LGBT%20Aging%20and%20Health%20Report_final.pdf. Accessed February 20, 2016.

Stigmatization

The physical and mental health disparities that exist today are rooted in and reflective of a long history of discrimination and bias against LGBTQ people, both at a societal level and within the health care system. Homosexuality was listed as a "Sociopathic Personality Disorder" in the American Psychiatric Institute's Diagnostic and Statistical Manual of Psychological Disorders as recently as the early 1970s. A transgender identity was listed in the Diagnostic and Statistical Manual of Psychological Disorders (DSM) as a psychological disorder as recently as 2013. As a consequence of the pathologizing of nonheterosexual sexual orientation and alternative gender identities, LGBTQ persons were sometimes subject to traumatizing medical interventions, such as castrations and electroshock therapy.[2]

Discrimination and abuse may not be as overt now, but it certainly still exists. Most LGBTQ people have encountered stigma and bias throughout their lives, and these experiences necessarily shape and affect how they interact with the health care system. This is particularly true for elderly LGBTQ people, who came of age when discrimination and dangerous stigmatization was more commonplace and codified into US laws and policies.[8] A comprehensive survey conducted in 2011 of LGBTQ older adults found that 82% of respondents had been victimized at least once in their lives as a result of their sexual orientation and/or gender identity.[1]

Social Supports

LGBTQ elders are twice as likely to live alone compared with their heterosexual peers, are more likely to be poor and isolated, and are three to four times less likely to have children that can help support them.[2] Research shows the LGBTQ older adults are more likely to feel unwelcome and actually be unwelcomed or mistreated in various health care settings, including nursing homes. The effects of this lack of social support and social isolation are detrimental. They include higher rates of depression, frequent hospitalizations, poverty, poor nutrition, delay in seeking medical care, and premature mortality.[2]

Advance Care Planning

Because LGBTQ elders are more likely to be estranged from their biological families, childless, and unmarried as they age, they tend to rely on what is known as "families of choice," friends and other community members who provide social connections and support.[2,3,9] Although these ties can be incredibly strong, institutional regulations and policies often do not recognize the legitimacy of these relationships. Families of choice and/or same-sex but unmarried partners are often denied the same rights and resources as legal spouses or biological family members.[2]

While same-sex marriage has recently been legalized in the United States, many LGBTQ persons are not partnered, and many partnered LGBTQ persons have not and will not choose to avail themselves of this right. Because laws regarding medical decision-making favor legal marriages and biological relationships, this can result in the unfortunate situation where an estranged biological family member's decision can override that of a same-sex partner or member of an LGBTQ patient's family of choice.[2,10]

In recent years, some states have passed legislation that has loosened restrictions regarding surrogate decision-making to allow domestic partners to act as health care proxies. For example, in 2010 New York passed the Family Health Care Decisions Act, which allows domestic partners or a "close adult friend" to act in the capacity of decision-maker as long as they are "familiar with the patient's personal, religious, and moral views regarding health care."[11] Although this is a step in the right direction, these laws vary from state to state, and LGBTQ people who reside in states with more progressive laws may not be aware of their rights.

Concerns About Disclosure

As a result of a long history of discrimination and the fear or expectation of substandard treatment, many LGBTQ people have reported that they are hesitant to reveal their sexual orientation or gender identity to their health care provider.[12] More than 20% reported that they did not disclose their sexual orientation or gender identity to their physician.[1] A review of the literature has shown that LGBTQ people are reluctant to "come out" to providers, and less likely to access health care services for fear of stigmatization.[11] When medical care is ultimately sought, worries about substandard treatment can also prevent or delay the disclosure of sexual orientation and/or gender identity to health care providers.[10] This lack of disclosure can lead to distress and compromised care.[13,14]

SPECIAL NEEDS OF THE TRANSGENDER POPULATION

The transgender and/or gender nonconforming population is a minority within a minority; it is estimated that only 0.3% of the adult population in the United States identifies as transgender.[1] As such, transgender people experience even more discrimination, stigma, and disparities than nearly any other minority group. They face serious obstacles and challenges when accessing health care, including primary care, and transgender-specific care.[15] It is estimated that up to 40% of transgender people do not have a regular health care provider, and tend to rely on emergency care and unsupervised self-care to meet their needs. Hormone therapy can confer many changes that are welcomed and desired by a transgender person. However, lack of adequate health care while taking exogenous hormones can confer increased health risks, as hormone therapy is associated with several physical and psychological complications. These complications include an increased risk of diabetes and cardiovascular disease, as well as liver and thromboembolic complications.[16] Although there is a dearth of research on this topic, it is reasonable to assume that any barriers to accessing palliative care experienced by the LGBTQ population are magnified in the transgender population.

NURSING IMPLICATIONS

Public attitudes and social policy that address how to best care for LGBTQ patients continues to evolve. The current palliative care experience of LGBTQ people is no longer primarily focused on caring for patients with HIV/AIDs. Although HIV/AIDS continues to be a major health issue, the aging LGBTQ population is dealing with a wider range of chronic illnesses, related to a variety of previously discussed risk factors.[3] In 2011, the Joint Commission instituted a new requirement for accreditation that mandated hospitals show specific evidence of how the unique needs of LGBTQ patients were being met.[17] Nursing is the largest workforce in the health care system, and are the providers that have the most frequent and close contact with patients and families. As such, nurses are well suited to spearhead the effort to address and meet these needs.

Stigmatization

A key obstacle to optimum end-of-life care for LGBTQ patients is decreased use of available resources that stems from fear of discrimination and a dearth of open, inclusive health care resources. This is a particularly sensitive issue for palliative care, because research has consistently shown that early palliative involvement can result in better outcomes, namely less depression, higher quality of life, and longer survival.[18,19] Heteronormativity, the presumption of heterosexuality as a given instead of one of several possible sexual orientations, and a lack of awareness of alternate gender identities, can result in a care environment that is unfriendly or even threatening to LGBTQ patients and family members.[20] Nurses can address the palliative care needs of LGBTQ patients by first examining current practice within their own institutions and agencies.

According to the Fenway Institute,[2] the first step to improving care for LGBTQ patients is to create an inclusive environment in all practices, including hospitals, nursing homes, and hospice agencies. Simple changes in signage, office and clinic environment, and intake or demographic forms that include nonstraight sexual orientation and alternative gender identities can make LGBTQ patients feel more comfortable and welcome. These changes should include prominent display of the institution's nondiscrimination policy, with specific mention of sexual orientation and gender identity.

Educational brochures on LGBTQ health topics can be made available where other patient information materials are displayed. The Joint Commission has recommended this and other approaches in a recently published field guide; this guide includes a self-assessment tool for clinicians or health care organizations seeking to become more inclusive.[21] A list of LGBTQ care resources is found in **Box 2**.

Disclosure

The decision to discuss sexual orientation and/or gender identity with health care providers is based on a patient's past experiences and possible negative reactions to disclosure.[22] Yet sexual orientation and gender identity are integral parts of a patient's social history. Their recognition and acceptance is an essential component of the provision of holistic, multidimensional, patient-centered palliative care. This is especially important when patients approach end-of-life and may need assistance in completing life review, achieving closure with loved ones, or conducting advance care planning. However, disclosure is a personal and individual process unique to each person's family and social circumstances. Clinicians should always be supportive, but not force the issue or pressure patients to speed the pace of this process.[2]

Open communication is key. Taking an open, nonjudgmental sexual and social history, that uses gender-neutral language, is integral to building trust with LGBTQ patients. Rather than making assumptions about sexual orientation or gender identity based on appearance or sexual behavior, clinicians should ask open-ended questions, mirroring the terms and pronouns patients use to describe themselves.[2] Questions should be framed in ways that allow patients to respond openly about their gender identity and/or sexual orientation and identify those who are most significant to them. Questions such as: "Who do you consider family/Who is family for you?" "Whom do you most rely on for support?" or "Do you currently have a significant other or partner?" open the door for an honest discussion of patient psychosocial supports and needs.[23] Clinicians may find that patients self-identify as more than one, or perhaps none of the LGBT labels. Some patients may instead identify as 'queer', an umbrella term that includes people who "(a) want to identify as queer and (b) who feel somehow outside of the societal norms in regards to gender and sexuality."[24] **Box 3** provides guidelines for communicating with LGBTQ patients.

Social Isolation and Limited Caregiver Availability

Discrimination in health care settings has been an issue for many LGBTQ persons, at times resulting in poor care or frank refusal of care.[10] Rawlings[4] describes how some

---

Box 2
Online resources

- Transgender Law Center's 10 Tips for Working with Transgender Individuals: A Guide for Health Care Providers. The Fenway Guide to Lesbian, Gay, Bisexual, and Transgender Health; Health Professionals Advancing LGBT Equality (http://www.glma.org)
- National Resource Center on LGBT Aging (http://lgbtagingcenter.org)
- National End of Life Care Programme. The Route to Success in End of Life Care - Achieving Quality for Lesbian, Gay, Bisexual and Transgender People (June 2012) (http://www.nhsiq.nhs.uk/resource-search/publications/eolc-rts-lgbt.aspx)
- SAGE: Services and Advocacy for Gay, Lesbian, Bisexual, and Transgender Elders (https://www.sageusa.org)
- Palliative Care Fast Facts: end-of-life and advance care planning considerations for lesbian, gay, bisexual, and transgender patient (https://www.mypcnow.org)
- Joint Commission: Checklists to Advance Effective Communication, Cultural Competence, and Patient- and Family-Centered Care for the Lesbian, Gay, Bisexual, and Transgender (LGBT) Community (http://www.jointcommission.org/assets/1/18/lgbtfieldguide.pdf)
- Joint Commission Field Guide to Advancing Effective Communication, Cultural Competence, and Patient- and Family-Centered Care for the Lesbian, Gay, Bisexual, and Transgender (LGBT) Community (http://www.jointcommission.org/assets/1/18/lgbtfieldguide.pdf)
- National Hospice Foundation: includes resources and educational webinars on LGBT end-of-life care (http://hospicefoundation.org/End-of-Life-Support-and-Resources/Coping-with-Terminal-Illness/How-to-Choose/LGBT-Resources)
- American Medical Association: Creating a Gay Friendly Practice. LGBT Resource Page (http://www.ama-assn.org/ama/pub/about-ama/our-people/member-groups-sections/glbt-advisory-committee/glbt-resources/create-lgbt-friendly-practice.page?)
- GLMA: Gay and Lesbian Medical Association Guidelines for Care of Lesbian, Gay, Bisexual and Transgender Patients (http://www.glma.org/_data/n_0001/resources/live/Welcoming%20Environment.pdf)
- Gen Silent (film about LGBT elders). Produced by Stu Maddux (http://gensilent.com/about-2/)
- Transgender Aging Network. Quick Tips for Caregivers of Transgender Clients. Nursing implications (http://forge-forward.org/wp-content/docs/caregiver_quicktips.pdf)

---

individuals may lead a dual life, living openly in some circles and not others. This can lead to significant stress when these worlds meet, in vulnerable moments, during periods of crisis, or at the end of life. Studies have shown that LGBTQ elders have few social supports and adult children to provide care in times of serious illness,[2,25] and hence may need to rely on professional caregivers. Mistrust of home health care providers may force LGBTQ patients back into the closet, their fear of exposure occurring even in their own home environment. Other end-of-life care situations are stressful for those who have not disclosed their sexual orientation. Partners of patients with dementia may fear that their confused loved ones may inadvertently "out them."[4] LGBTQ partners may also feel vulnerable when leaving their loved ones in hospitals or nursing homes where staff members are perceived as homophobic.[26] Hospice and palliative care nurses must be particularly cognizant of their own personal attitudes and how they approach LGBTQ patients in these especially sensitive times. It is important to raise staff awareness of these issues, and conduct ongoing meetings with open discussion of personal perspectives and staff values. Potentially harmful attitudes and biased beliefs should be re-evaluated and resolved as much as possible. Patient advocates should be available and visible, as safe supports and institutional

---

Box 3
Guidelines for open communication

1. Use neutral and inclusive language in interviews and when talking with all patients

2. Keep an open mind; avoid assumptions about a person's sexual orientation or gender identity based on appearance.

3. Unsure of a person's orientation or identity: use gender-neutral language to ask: "How would you like to be addressed?" or "What name would you like to be called?"

4. Sexual identity and behavior are only one part of a person's identity. Also assess family relationships, religion, class, socioeconomic status, beliefs, race, ethnicity, ability/disability

5. Be mindful of language that assumes heterosexuality.
   a. Avoid "Are you married?" or references to husbands/wives.
   b. Instead ask, "Do you have a partner or a significant other?"

6. Assess and as appropriate, use the patient's' own wording, terms, and language when describing their own sexual orientation and their relationships.

7. Respect an individual's right to disclose information at their own pacing and choice.

From The White House Office of the Press Secretary. Presidential Memorandum - Hospital Visitation. Available at: https://www.whitehouse.gov/the-press-office/presidential-memorandum-hospital-visitation.

---

ambassadors for LGBTQ patients. Outward signs of openness, as simple as rainbow symbols on display, can provide reassurance that staff have received education and are part of an "LBGTQ friendly" organization. The American Medical Association and the Gay and Lesbian Medical Association provide specific recommendations for practice organization and staff training, which can assist in educating all staff on these crucial issues (see resources in **Box 2**).

Transgender People at High Risk

Transgender people are likely to have been victims of sexual violence, hate crimes, and abuse at some point in their life.[27] There is very little research focused specifically on the attitudes toward and issues facing transgender people. Most studies have included transgender issues, lumped together in more general LGBTQ research. A recent review of psychosocial literature on transgender elders[27] found that this population has significant concerns about facing discrimination, potential abuse at the hands of caregivers, an inability to live openly at the end of life. They also expressed fears regarding loss of independence, the threat of becoming homeless, and loss of mental capacity. One study that surveyed a cohort of 276 older-adult transgender people who also identified as lesbians found that most had significant fears about potential late-life illness, end-of-life care, and legal issues stemming from their transgender identity.[27] At end of life, painful life review and posttraumatic stress disorder may surface; educated and aware nurses can recognize these psychological issues, address anxiety, and facilitate appropriate referrals. The large scale (n = 1963) Trans MetLife Survey on Later-Life Preparedness and Perceptions in Transgender-identified Individuals revealed even more disturbing data: because of fear of how they would be treated, a subset of respondents reported either pondering or already having plans for suicide when faced with deteriorating health status.[28] Vigilant and caring assessments of psychological and spiritual distress are a nursing imperative. Above all, nurses have a crucial responsibility to ensure a safe environment for these patients at the end of life, a time when they are most vulnerable.

LGBTQ Elders at High Risk

There may be generational differences among LGBTQ persons regarding comfort and openness in divulging information about sexual orientation or gender identity in health care settings. Openness about sexuality and sexual orientation has changed over time, but historical events (eg, past classification of homosexuality as a mental illness) have left a legacy of distrust for many older LGBTQ persons.[4] Compared with younger people for whom sexual diversity may seem more common and acceptable, older LGBTQ persons may have experienced more intense discrimination over time. This could predispose them to increased reluctance to disclose information to care providers.[3] Readers are encouraged to view the film, "Gen Silent," for a poignant portrayal of six LGBTQ elders facing health issues and decisions.[29]

Care of "Families of Choice"

In many cases, LGBTQ persons make distinctions between "families of origin" (biological family) and "families of choice."[3] Historically, unmarried partners have often been left out of medical decisions and opportunities to provide care and comfort to their loved ones. In 2010, President Obama issued a presidential memorandum addressing this issue, clearly articulating the heart-wrenching circumstances experienced by some LGBTQ patients and their partners (**Box 4**).

In response to this presidential memorandum, the Centers for Medicare and Medicaid Services made changes to policy regarding hospital visitation. The new mandate required hospitals to include visitation rights within its patient bill of rights. Notably, the final rule makes it clear that Medicare and Medicaid participating hospitals may not restrict, limit, or otherwise deny visitation privileges based on sexual orientation or gender identity.[2]

Further progress has been made recently in advancing the rights of LGBTQ patients and their 'families of choice' across many domains, including health care. Most notable is the 2015 Supreme Court ruling that repealed the Defense of Marriage Act and legalized marriage for same-sex couples.[30] Patients, families, and professionals alike must be knowledgeable about these recent rulings and patient rights. This recent legal progress does not preclude the importance of clearly considered and

---

Box 4
Excerpt from Presidential Memorandum on Hospital Visitation, 2010

...uniquely affected are gay and lesbian Americans who are often barred from the bedsides of the partners with whom they may have spent decades of their lives— unable to be there for the person they love, and unable to act as a legal surrogate if their partner is incapacitated. For all of these Americans, the failure to have their wishes respected concerning who may visit them or make medical decisions on their behalf has real consequences. It means that doctors and nurses do not always have the best information about patients' medications and medical histories and that friends and certain family members are unable to serve as intermediaries to help communicate patients' needs. It means that a stressful and at times terrifying experience for patients is senselessly compounded by indignity and unfairness. And it means that all too often, people are made to suffer or even to pass away alone, denied the comfort of companionship in their final moments while a loved one is left worrying and pacing down the hall.

From The Joint Commission. Advancing effective communication, cultural competence, and patient- and family centered care for the lesbian, gay, bisexual, and transgender (LGBT) community: a field guide. Oak Brook (IL): JCAHO; 2011; with permission.

documented advance directives, because the full impact of this legislation has yet to be determined.[3]

IMPLICATIONS FOR NURSING EDUCATION

A recent review of baccalaureate nursing education revealed that serious deficits in addressing LGBTQ issues exist in nursing curricula nationwide.[31] There is a need to better define the cultural competencies required to best meet the needs of the LGBTQ population to subsequently develop associated educational programs across inter-professional programs.[3] Values clarification and appropriate attitude adjustment should occur early in one's professional education. Lim and Bernstein[31] recommend use of trained live actors in simulation laboratories to present realistic, standardized, and replicable learning scenarios. Nursing faculty have a mandate to review and revise curricular content to better address LGBTQ palliative care. Content mapping and ongoing faculty development can lead to better integration of LGBTQ care, incorporating this essential information into lectures, assignments, and clinical opportunities.

IMPLICATIONS FOR NURSING POLICY

Many LGBTQ people live alone without adequate services. Nurses can work to help forge a partnership between existing general LGBTQ services available in the community and needed health services. Health care systems must develop public health initiatives aimed at this high-risk target population. The overall aims should be to reduce the risk of developing chronic disease (ie, programs to address obesity, alcohol abuse, and smoking) and to continue to support and expand programs that address HIV prevention, education, and treatment. LGBTQ-specific programs should be expanded to include elder-specific services, health advocacy, and advance care planning. Community input from direct stakeholders is invaluable in informing the development of agency programs and policies. As holistic care providers, nurses should be fully aware of the multidimensional nature of care and actively contribute to this kind of program development.

IMPLICATIONS FOR NURSING RESEARCH

Research on aging and palliative care should include sexual orientation and gender identity measures, to further define risk, mortality, and morbidity. At the same time, it is important to avoid the error of lumping LGBTQ persons together into a single sexual minority, when there likely exists significant heterogeneity among the sub-groups in terms of health issues, attitudes, and practices. Future palliative care studies are needed to analyze life and illness trajectories in these specific populations, end-of-life decision-making practices, and availability and use of supports. Best practices in nursing education can develop future generations of nurses to meet the ongoing needs of LGBTQ patients.

SUMMARY

The increasing amount of research and published professional reflection highlight the need for special focus on the palliative care needs of LGBTQ patients. Nursing has long been considered among the most trusted professions, and as such, can reach this vulnerable minority and positively impact the quality of care provided to LGBTQ patients.

As with all patient populations, effectively serving LGBTQ patients requires clinicians to understand the cultural context of their patients' lives, and modify practice policies and environments to be inclusive. By taking comprehensive and nonjudgmental histories, educating themselves about appropriate and unique health issues, and reflecting on personal attitudes that might inhibit optimal care, nurses can provide compassionate and professional care to LGBTQ people. The very nature of palliative care affirms the unique value and perspectives of all people, and can best address the multidimensional nature of health issues faced by LGBTQ people with serious, advanced illness.

REFERENCES

1. Fredriksen-Goldsen KI, Kim HJ, Emlet CA, et al. The aging in health report: disparities and resilience among lesbian, gay, bisexual, and transgender older adults. Institute for Multigenerational Health. 2011. Available at: http://www.lgbtagingcenter.org/resources/pdfs/LGBT%20Aging%20and%20Health%20Report_final.pdf. Accessed February 20, 2016.
2. Ard KL, Makdon HJ. Improving the health care of lesbian, gay, bisexual, and transgender (LGBT) People. Boston (MA): The Fenway Institute; 2012. Available at: http://www.lgbthealtheducation.org/wp-content/uploads/12-054_LGBTHealtharticle_v3_07-09-12.pdf.
3. Griebling TL. Sexuality and aging: a focus on lesbian, gay, bisexual and transgender (LGBT) needs in palliative and end of life care. Curr Opin Support Palliat Care 2016;10:95–101.
4. Rawlings D. End-of-life care considerations for gay, lesbian, bisexual, and transgender individuals. Int J Palliat Nurs 2012;18:29–34.
5. Cochran SD, Mays VM. Burden of psychiatric morbidity among lesbian, gay and bisexual individuals in the California Quality of Life Survey. J Abnorm Psychol 2009;118:647–58.
6. Rothman EF, Exner D, Baughman A. The prevalence of sexual assault against people who identify as gay, lesbian or bisexual in the United States: a systematic review. Trauma Violence Abuse 2011;12:55–66.
7. Mutanski B, Andrews R, Puckett JA. The effects of cumulative victimization on mental health among lesbian, gay, bisexual, and transgender adolescents and young adults. Am J Public Health 2016;106:527–33.
8. Committee on Lesbian, Gay, Bisexual, and Transgender Health Issues and Research Gaps and Opportunities, Context for LGBT health status in the United States, Institute of Medicine. The health of lesbian, gay, bisexual, and transgender people: building a foundation for better understanding. Washington, DC: National Academies Press (US); 2011. p. 25–88.
9. Hash KM, Netting FE. Long-term planning and decision-making among midlife and older gay men and lesbians. J Soc Work End Life Palliat Care 2007;3:59–77.
10. Harding R, Epiphaniou E, Chidgey-Clark J. Needs, experiences, and preferences of sexual minorities for end-of-life care and palliative care: a systematic review. J Palliat Med 2012;15:602–11.
11. Goldfarb D. New York's Family Health Care Decisions Act. Available at: http://www.seniorlaw.com/new-yorks-family-health-care-decisions-act-4/. Accessed February 21, 2016.
12. Eliason MJ, Schope R. Does "Don't ask don't tell" apply to health care? lesbian, gay, and bisexual people's disclosure to health care providers. J Gay Lesb Med Assoc 2001;5:125–34.
13. Facione NC, Facione PA. Perceived prejudice in healthcare and women's health protective behavior. Nurs Res 2007;56:175–84.

14. Lick DJ, Durso LE, Johnson KL. Minority stress and physical health among sexual minorities. Perspect Psychol Sci 2013;8:521–48.

15. Bauer GR, Hammand R, Travers R, et al. I don't think this is theoretical; This is our lives: how erasure impacts health care for transgender people. J Assoc Nurses AIDS Care 2009;20:348–61.

16. Williams ME, Freeman PA. Transgender health: Implications for aging and caregiving. J Gay Lesb Soc Serv 2007;18:93–108.

17. Lim F, Pace JC, Bailey K, et al. Caring for older gay lesbian bisexual and transgender adults. Amer Nurs Today 2013. Available at: http://www.americannursetoday.com/caring-for-older-lesbian-gay-bisexual-and-transgender-adults/. Accessed February 12, 2016.

18. Bakitas M, Doyle KD, Hegel MT, et al. Effects of a palliative care intervention on clinical outcomes in patients with advanced cancer: the Project ENABLE II randomized control trial. J Amer Med Assoc 2009;302:741–9.

19. Temel JS, Greer JA, Muzikansky A. Early palliative care for patients with metastatic non-small-cell lung cancer. N Engl J Med 2010;363:733–42.

20. Cartwright C, Hughes M, Leinert T. End–of-life care for gay, lesbian, bisexual, and transgender people. Cult Health Sex 2012;14(5):537–48.

21. The Joint Commission. Advancing effective communication, cultural competence, and patient- and family centered care for the lesbian, gay, bisexual, and transgender (LGBT) community: a field guide. Oak Brook (IL): JCAHO; 2011.

22. Boehmer U, Case P. Physicians don't ask, sometimes patients tell: disclosure of sexual orientation among women with breast cancer. Cancer 2004;101:1182–9.

23. Lawton A, White J, Fromme E. End-of-life and advance care planning considerations for lesbian, gay, bisexual, and transgender patient. Fast facts and concepts. 2014; 275. Available at: http://www.mypcnow.org. Accessed January 30, 2016.

24. A definition of 'queer'. PFLAG (Parents and Families of Lesbians and Gays) Website. 2016. Available at: https://community.pflag.org/abouttheq. Accessed February 29, 2016.

25. Rivera E, Wilson SR, Jennings LK. Long-term care and life planning preferences for older gays and lesbians. J Ethnograph Qual Res 2011;5:157–70.

26. Brotman S, Ryan B, Cormier R. Coming out to care: caregivers of gay and lesbian seniors in Canada. Gerontologist 2007;47:490–503.

27. Witten TM. Elder transgender lesbians: exploring the intersection of age, lesbian sexual identity, and transgender identity. J Lesbian Stud 2015;19:73–89.

28. Witten TM. It's not all darkness: robustness, resilience, and successful transgender aging. LGBT Health 2014;1:24–33.

29. Maddux S. Gen silent 2010. Available at: http://gensilent.com/about-2/. Accessed February 18, 2016.

30. Wahlert L, Fiester A. A false sense of security: lesbian, gay, bisexual and transgender (LGBT) surrogate health care decision-making rights. J Am Board Fam Med 2013;26:802–4.

31. Lim FA, Bernstein I. Promoting awareness of LGBT issues in aging in a baccalaureate nursing program. Nurs Educ Perspect 2012;33:170–5.

Palliative Wound Care for Malignant Fungating Wounds

Holistic Considerations at End-of-Life

Charles Tilley, MS, ANP-BC, ACHPN, CWOCN[a,b,c],*,
Jana Lipson, RN, BA, BSN[d], Mark Ramos, RN, BSN[e]

KEYWORDS

- Malignant fungating wound • Fungating wounds • Malignant wounds • Odor
- Symptoms • Qualitative • Psychological • Quality of life

KEY POINTS

- A holistic approach is essential to caring for people with malignant fungating wounds (MFWs) because they suffer from a devastating and often crippling physical symptom burden that may subsequently lead to spiritual and psychosocial distress with diminished quality of life.
- A comprehensive patient- and family-centered care planning approach at end-of-life includes PALCARE: *P*rognosis, *A*dvance care planning, *L*iving situation, *C*omprehensive history, *A*ssessment, evidence-based *R*ecommendations and *E*ducation of patient, family and staff.
- Interventions aimed at easing the suffering of terminally ill people with MFWs should be realistic and based on the best available evidence, balancing respect for goals of care with available resources.
- The complexity of caring for patients with MFWs necessitates specialist-level guidance by a wound, ostomy, and continence nurse (WOCN) preferably with a palliative care background and certification in the hospice and palliative care specialty (CHPN, ACHPN).

INTRODUCTION: THE MAGNITUDE OF SUFFERING

Malignant fungating wounds (MFWs) afflict 5% of patients with advanced cancers[1] and 10% of patients with metastasis[2] with life expectancy averaging 6 to 12 months.[2–4]

Conflict of Interest: The authors disclose no conflict of interest.
[a] International Advanced Practice Palliative Care Partners, LLC, New York, NY 10014, USA; [b] New York University College of Nursing, New York, NY 10016, USA; [c] VNSNY Hospice and Palliative Care, New York, NY 10001, USA; [d] Observation Unit, NYU Langone Medical Center, New York, NY 10016, USA; [e] Medical-Surgical Unit, Northwell Lenox Hill Hospital, New York, NY 10075, USA
* Corresponding author.
E-mail address: tillec01@nyu.edu

Nurs Clin N Am 51 (2016) 513–531
http://dx.doi.org/10.1016/j.cnur.2016.05.006   **nursing.theclinics.com**
0029-6465/16/$ – see front matter © 2016 Elsevier Inc. All rights reserved.

Unfortunately, no population-based cancer register records the incidence of MFWs,[5] and prevalence is underreported because of shame, embarrassment, and fear,[6] thus a more precise estimate is currently impossible. Incidence is anticipated to increase rapidly as the number of new cancer cases in the aging population rises with people living longer because of significant innovations in treatment. Because MFWs are managed primarily through palliative wound care approaches and most of these patients do not survive, it is realistic to project that more and more people with MFWs will enter hospice programs. Developing a pragmatic, patient- and family-centered palliative wound care plan is a key to alleviating suffering.

MFWs have been referred to in the literature by multiple names using interchangeable terms.[7,8] MFWs are defined by Grocott[9] as the infiltration and proliferation of malignant cells in to the skin and its supporting blood and lymph vessels. "Fungating" is described by Mortimer[10] as infiltration and erosion through the skin by a proliferation of malignant tumor cells ultimately causing ulceration. MFWs may result from primary tumors or secondary lesions (metastasis) (**Fig. 1**).[11] MFWs of the breast and head and neck are by far the most prevalent (**Box 1**).

The root of suffering in this population is based largely in physical symptom distress; excruciating and debilitating pain, unbearable pruritus, malodor, excessive exudates, and unpredictable bleeding resulting in psychological anguish, shame, humiliation, loss of confidence, fear, guilt, depression, anxiety, and social isolation.[3,4,12,13] The devastating effects of MFWs on quality of life have also been described.[14,15]

Most early publications and research emphasize physical description and management of symptoms. Interventional research in the area of MFWs has remained sparse, with a recent Cochrane Review of topical agents and dressings for MFWs finding the evidence base negligible.[5] This dearth of research presents a multitude of challenges to practitioners.

The cases of Ms. C and Ms. A are used to introduce the PALCARE mnemonic (*P*rognosis, *A*dvance care planning, *L*iving situation, *C*omprehensive history, *A*ssessment, evidence-based *R*ecommendations and *E*ducation of patient, family and staff) (**Box 2**) as a framework for developing a holistic, systematic, patient-centered

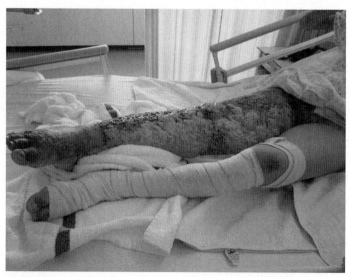

Fig. 1. MFW of entire right leg with lymphedema from metastatic colon cancer.

Box 1
MFW incidence by location

Breast	62%
Head and neck	24%
Genitalia	3%
Back	3%
Other site	8%

Data from Lo S, Hu W, Hayter M, et al. Experiences of living with a malignant fungating wound: a qualitative study. J Clin Nurs 2008;17(20):2700.

Box 2
A systematic approach: PALCARE

- Prognosis
  - Hospice diagnosis and Palliative Performance Score
  - Is the patient's life expectancy weeks or months?
  - Is the patient in the last hours or days of life?

- Advance care planning
  - Goals of care
    - Further hospitalizations
    - Resuscitation wishes: full code status versus natural death
    - Antibiotics: intravenous, oral, topical
    - Artificial nutrition or hydration
    - Emergency management clarification (hemorrhage, sepsis)

- Living situation
  - Caregiver availability
  - Caregiver participation (willingness)
  - Caregiver ability (cognitive/physical)
  - Caregiver reliability
  - Environment/setting (running water, shower)
  - Consider appropriate hospice level of care
    - Inpatient hospice (IPU) for uncontrolled symptoms
    - Hospice home care (symptoms manageable in the community)

- Comprehensive history
  - Review of symptoms, activities of daily living, complementary alternative medicine
  - Wound and associated symptoms (pain, pruritus odor, exudates, bleeding, number of dressing changes, current dressing plan)
  - Psychiatric (Patient Health Questionnaire 2, Generalized Anxiety Disorder 7)
  - Social (legal status, insurance, employment, fiduciary/housing/food insecurity)
  - Spiritual (FICA tool)

- Assessment
  - Comprehensive assessment
  - Focused wound assessment
  - Wound photographs (follow institution policy)
  - Wound cultures, laboratory studies (as necessary)

- Recommendations
  - Establish symptom management priorities (pain, pruritus, odor, exudates, bleeding) and palliative wound care goals
  - Topical and/or systemic interventions
  - Referrals: wound, ostomy, and continence nurse (if not already involved), psychiatry, spiritual care, and so forth

- Education
  - Patient, family, caregivers
  - Staff education
    - Hospice medical directors, administrators, wound care resource nurses

palliative wound care approach in end-of-life care. **Figs. 2** and **3** include the first three steps to the PALCARE method: *Prognosis, Advance* care planning, and *Living* situation.

ROLE OF THE HOSPICE AND PALLIATIVE CARE WOUND, OSTOMY, AND CONTINENCE NURSE

Wound, ostomy, and continence nursing, formally recognized by the American Nurses Association in 2010 as a nursing specialty,[16] has evolved from its inception in 1961 as an enterostomal therapist education program to what is known today as the Wound, Ostomy and Continence Nurses Society.[17] National certification may be obtained at either the baccalaureate or graduate level.[17]

The need for expert help is a theme that emerges from the qualitative literature. In a descriptive study by Lo and colleagues,[3] patients with MFWs and their caregivers voiced expectations that specialist-level wound care would be available at the onset of their illness. Unfortunately, lack of access to this care was consistent across settings, leaving patients to improvise strategies with little or no expert guidance. This led to anxiety, lack of confidence, and social isolation.[3] These authors recommend every hospice program employ or consult with a certified wound, ostomy, and continence nurse ideally certified in hospice and palliative care (CHPN, ACHPN). Dual certification ensures a level of expertise in caring for those with advanced illness requiring palliative wound, ostomy, and continence services and allows nursing professionals to practice under the full scope of their licensure in the palliative care setting, as outlined in **Box 3**.

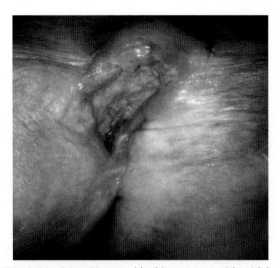

Fig. 2. Vaginal MFW. *P*: Ms. C is a 57-year-old white woman with widely metastatic vulvar cancer status post vulvectomy, radiation, and chemotherapy. She has a life expectancy of 2 to 3 weeks and a Palliative Performance Score of 30%. *A*: She is do not resuscitate/do not intubate, declines hospitalization or heroic measures, and will accept oral and/or topical antibiotics. *L*: She is transferred to the hospice inpatient unit from home with uncontrolled pain, malodor, and excessive exudates from a vaginal MFW. She was self-managing the wound with obstetric pads, showers, and frequent changes of underwear and pants when soiled. Her primary caregiver is overwhelmed and unable to care for her at home.

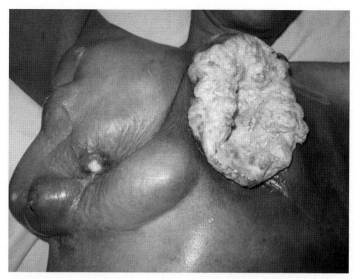

Fig. 3. Breast MFW. *P*: Ms. A is a 52-year-old African American woman with metastatic breast cancer status post left mastectomy, radiation, and chemotherapy. Her life expectancy is 2 to 3 months, and Palliative Performance Score is 50%. *A*: She is a do not resuscitate/do not intubate; declines hospitalization or heroic measures; and will accept intravenous, oral, and/or topical antibiotics. *L*: She presented to the hospice inpatient unit with fevers, chills, malodor, excessive exudates, and uncontrolled periwound pain and pruritus from a breast MFW. She describes herself as "living in her bathroom" for the last 3 weeks, changing dressings every 2 hours, has no primary caregiver, and does not believe she can manage at home anymore.

PSYCHOSOCIAL ASPECTS OF CARE

Lawton,[19] during her 10-month observational study of hospice patients enduring horrific physical and psychological suffering, introduced the concept of being "unbounded." The state of becoming unbounded was caused by odors, exudates, pain, bleeding, and disfigurement as a result of "the disintegrating, decaying body," with the dying experiencing marginalization, isolation, and loss of self and social identity.[19] Her study notably included patients with fungating tumors of the head and neck, groin and genitalia, and breast.

Phenomenologic studies provide additional, often painful insights into the psychological and spiritual suffering of patients with MFWs. The gruesome and often unpredictable nature of their symptoms, combined with the time-consuming demands of wound care, robs these patients of their dignity, confidence, and even relationships. Symptom distress also impacts significantly on activities of daily living and has been shown to decrease overall quality of life.[15,20]

Nonacceptance of limited prognosis leads some to use denial as a coping mechanism and avoid seeking treatment of their wounds or evaluation of their feelings. Disfiguring lesions are a constant reminder of disease, leading to feelings of hopelessness. At times this results in downplaying distress, independently treating their symptoms or in the extreme, even neglecting their wounds entirely. Some experts link the development of personality disorders, anxiety, and depression to the relentless sequelae of cancer and impending death.[12,13] However, the presence of a malignant wound was found at times to cause more psychological suffering than the cancer diagnosis itself.[21]

Box 3
Role of the hospice and palliative care wound, ostomy, and continence nurse

Educator

- Patient and caregiver education
- Staff education
- Profession education at the local, national, and international level

Consultant

- Specialist-level wound, ostomy, and continence intra-agency consultation
- Specialist-level consultation to outside or referring agencies
- Chair of the hospice and palliative care wound, ostomy, and continence nurse committee

Researcher

- Conducts or participates in research based on the National Institute for Nursing Research: Palliative Care Research Foci, 2011[18]
  - Palliative and end-of-life care
  - Quality of life: symptom management initiatives
- Promotes evidence-based nursing

Administrator

- Wound, ostomy, and continence supply management
  - Cost analysis and containment
  - Formulary development
  - Product evaluation
- Continuous quality improvement
  - Patient satisfaction
  - Pressure ulcer prevalence and incidence
  - Wound registry for MFW prevalence
- Policy, procedure, and protocol development

Body image has a great impact on psychological well-being because it is associated with one's identity. Studies on femininity demonstrate a loss of confidence among women with MFWs. Because of the breast's connection with sexuality and being female, women report feeling less attractive and avoid intimacy with their partners.[22] Furthermore, women report feeling mutilated and disgusted by their wounds, as though they are witnessing their bodies decompose.[23] As a result, these individuals feel as though they have lost control over their lives and are marginalized, subsequently withdrawing from society.[4,13,22]

The hospice team uses timely screening, assessment, interventions, and referrals in addressing these psychosocial issues. Depression and anxiety screening tools, such as the Patient Health Questionnaire 2 (**Box 4**) and Generalized Anxiety Disorder 7 (**Box 5**), should be used to identify patients at risk for depression and anxiety and allow for timely interventions and referrals. The authors recommend screening on entry into the hospice program, at least every 2 to 4 weeks thereafter, and with each contact by the hospice nurse practitioner or hospice medical director. Decisions to refer to a licensed clinical social worker (LCSW) or psychologist for counseling or a psychiatrist for evaluation and pharmacologic recommendations should be a shared-decision with the patient and family.

Box 4
Patient Health Questionnaire 2

1. Over the past 2 weeks, have you felt down, depressed, or hopeless?

2. Over the past 2 weeks, have you felt little interest or pleasure in doing things?

From Pfizer. Patient Health Questionnaire screeners. Available at: http://www.phqscreeners. com. Accessed February 23, 2016.

Financial stability should be explored because many patients and their caregivers are incapable of working due to the limitations of their illness.[4] Investigation of housing and/or food insecurity may be undertaken by social work. Hospice programs cover the cost of dressing supplies, durable medical equipment, and medications related to the hospice diagnosis.

PSYCHOSOCIAL ASPECTS OF CARE: COMPLEMENTARY ALTERNATIVE MEDICINE

The role of complementary alternative medicine (CAM) in the holistic care of MFWs is promising, although research is limited. Therapies found in **Box 6** as CAM have been shown to decrease suffering and improve overall well-being.[4] Research in the area of CAM ranges from expert opinion; case reports; and small, nonrandomized qualitative studies. Guided imagery and meditation may also prove to be therapeutic, although no studies to date examine these techniques in patients with MFWs.

SPIRITUAL ASPECTS OF CARE

Suffering and limited prognosis cause patients to consider their own mortality[29] and review their existential beliefs and connection to spirituality. Loss of hope may occur as the fungating wound grows in size, new lesions appear, or new symptoms emerge.[13,23] Patients regularly make reference to faith, to include those not previously identified as spiritual or religious.[4] The FICA tool (*F*aith and beliefs, *I*mportance, *C*ommunity, *A*ddress in care) is used to screen patients' spiritual beliefs on admission.[30] Referral to pastoral care is recommended if risk for existential distress is

---

Box 5
Generalized Anxiety Disorder 7

Over the last 2 weeks, how often have you been bothered by the following problems?

1. Feeling nervous, anxious, or on edge

2. Not being able to stop or control worrying

3. Worrying too much about different things

4. Trouble relaxing

5. Being so restless that it's hard to sit still

6. Becoming easily annoyed or irritable

7. Feeling afraid as if something awful might happen

From Pfizer. Patient Health Questionnaire screeners. Available at: http://www.phqscreeners. com. Accessed February 23, 2016.

Box 6
CAM interventions

- Massage and touch therapy
- Music therapy
- Aromatherapy
- Occupational therapy

Data from Refs.[24–28]

---

identified. The hospice team should be sensitive to and supportive of all religious and spiritual beliefs.

PHYSICAL ASPECTS OF CARE: PAIN

Pain associated with MFWs has multiple etiologies, detrimental effects on quality of life,[14,15] and is a common distressing complaint.[3,12,20,23] The skin has the most sensory nerve endings of any organ in the body and has special nociceptors that can perceive mechanical, thermal, or chemical injury, which may be somatic, neuropathic, or mixed in nature.[31] **Box 7** lists pathologic and iatrogenic causes of temporary (incident) and persistent pain (between dressing changes, at night, and at rest).[32]

Comprehensive pain assessments are guided by the total pain concept, which includes physical, psychological, spiritual, and social factors.[35] Pain in advanced cancer is one of the most common and distressing symptoms reported. Pain assessment must include wound- and nonwound-related pain or discomfort and exploration of temporary and persistent wound pain etiologies, and use of a valid and reliable tool is recommended. The total pain approach (**Box 8**) includes symptom management for malignancy-related pain, interdisciplinary involvement to address psychosocial or spiritual factors, and specialist-level wound care for local discomfort.

Box 7
Etiology of pain

Pathologic

- Direct tumor compression of an organ
- Dermal erosion and exposure of nerve endings
- Damage of nerves related to direct tumor invasion or compression
- Edema secondary to impaired lymphatic or drainage, or wound infection

Iatrogenic

- Manipulation of dressings
- Inappropriate dressing selection
- Adhesives
- Wound cleansing or irrigation
- Debridement

Data from Refs.[32–34]

Box 8
Total pain management

Total pain origin

- Physical factors
  - Malignancy pain
    - Somatic, neuropathic, or mixed
  - Wound care
    - Vigorous irrigation or rubbing of fragile tissue with cleansing
    - Frequent dressing manipulation and changes
    - Adherence of dressings to the to the wound bed during dressing removal
    - Painful wound bed
  - Infection
  - Medical adhesive-related skin injury

- Psychological and social factors
  - Housing, food, fiduciary insecurities
  - Anxiety, depression, grief and prebereavement issues
  - Body image disturbances

- Spiritual factors
  - Existential angst

Interventions and referrals

- Long-acting opioids, short-acting breakthrough opioids, adjuvant pharmacologic and nonpharmacological interventions per nurse practitioner or hospice medical director

- Gentle irrigation, patting or blotting of wound bed

- Decrease number of changes with moisture-retentive dressings

- Soaking dressing before removal with normal saline (NS) or tepid tap water

- Nonadherent dressings: foams, petrolatum-based, silicone

- Topical opioids (10 mg morphine in 8 g hydrogel)[36]

- Topical anesthetics (2% lidocaine jelly 3–5 minutes before wound care)[36]

- Antimicrobial dressings and/or systemic antibiotics

- Use of burn net or garments, such as postsurgical bras, Lycra, or Attends undergarments to secure dressings

- If adhesives are necessary use skin protectants and apply paper tape

- Referral to social work, grief counselor

- Use of garments, such as Dale bras or Attends undergarments, to secure dressings and normalize body image (**Fig. 4**)

- Referral to spiritual care

Adapted from Walsh A, Bradley M, Cavallito K. Management of fungating tumors and pressure ulcers in a patient with stage IV cutaneous malignant melanoma. J Hosp Palliat Nurs 2014;16(4):208–14.

PHYSICAL ASPECTS OF CARE: ODOR AND EXUDATES

"Garbage," "rotting flesh," and "cadavers" are descriptors elicited from patients, family members, and other caregivers (including nurses) when asked to describe the malodor from MFWs.[3,20] The characteristic smell is attributed to proliferation of aerobic and anaerobic bacteria, the latter of which thrives in oxygen-free necrotic tissue found in fungating wound beds. Malodor has often been cited as

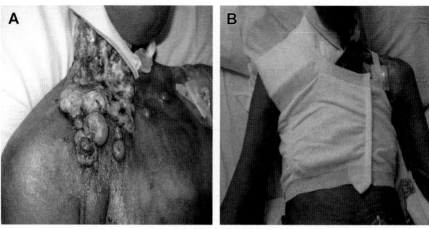

Fig. 4. Fungating wound of head and neck extending to right chest wall before (*A*) and after (*B*) dressing change secured with Dale bra.

the most distressing symptom to patients and caregivers because the odor may be pervasive, permeating the clothes of the patient, caregivers, and staff alike; linens; furniture; and even escaping into hallways, defying the boundaries of a hospice room.

Topical antimicrobial therapy and absorbent dressings, combined with cleansing and odor-eliminating interventions, have been the mainstay of MFW odor and exudate treatment. Despite multiple studies, a Cochrane Review[5] identified only one randomized control trial by Kalemikerakis[37] that provided weak evidence suggesting silver foam dressings may reduce malodor.[5] The effect of topical antimicrobial dressings on microbial resistance, biofilms, and the characterization of microbiomes in MFWs is also largely unknown. **Table 1** lists select interventions that may be used to control odor and exudates.

PHYSICAL ASPECTS OF CARE: MOISTURE-ASSOCIATED SKIN DAMAGE AND PRURITUS

Periwound moisture-associated dermatitis is one of four subcategories included under the umbrella term moisture-associated skin damage (MASD) and is a key consideration in the care of patients with MFWs. Heavily exudating wounds may cause an overhydration of the skin and maceration, leading to further skin breakdown, infections, pain, or pruritus.[41] Maceration of the skin is described as irritation and damage of the skin adjacent (within a 4-cm periwound border) to a wound caused by supersaturation.[42] The bordering skin may present as maceration; pale, white, or gray wrinkled skin[43] or inflammation; erythema; and swelling, usually associated with pain or pruritus. **Fig. 5** demonstrates circumferential irritation and pronounced swelling and erythema from 2 o'clock to 6 o'clock, which was caused by heavy exudates without the use of absorptive dressings or periwound skin protection.

Composition of exudates, in addition to volume, has been shown to correlate with risk of developing MASD.[44] One study of 20 women with fungating breast wounds found exudates with higher levels of putrescine and with the presence of cadaverine were associated with higher incidence of periwound moisture-associated dermatitis and pruritus.[45]

Table 1
Dressings and antibacterial agents to control odor and drainage

Dressings and Antibacterial Agents	Examples of Brands	Beneficial Effects and Considerations	Cost
Foams	• Allevyn (Smith & Nephew) • Aquacel Foam (Convatec) • Tegaderm Foam (3M) • Mepilex (Monlynlycke Health Care)	Promotes moist wound environment and does not adhere to tissue. Prevents strikethrough. Multiple shapes and sizes available to fit difficult dressing sites (ie, heels) and conforms to the body.	• 5 × 5 box = $$ • 5 × 5 box = $$ • 6 × 6 box = $$ • 6 × 6 box = $$
Calcium alginates	• Algicell (Derma Sciences) • Algisite M (Smith & Nephew) • Tegaderm High Gelling (3M)	May be used to cover or fill wound bed. Dressing material becomes a gel and absorbs any drainage while promoting a moist wound bed. May act as a hemostatic agent.	• 4 × 4 box = $ • 4 × 4 box = $ • 4 × 4 box = $
Honey	• Activon Tulle (Avancis) • Medihoney (Medihoney)	Supersaturated sugar solution with high osmolarity, low water activity. Bactericidal, moistens wound and removes necrotic tissue. Lowers wound pH to promote healing.	• 4 × 4 box = $ • 4 × 4 box = $
Silver	• Aquacel Ag hydrofiber (Convatec) • Acticoat 3 (Smith & Nephew) • Optifoam Ag (Medline)	Gradual release of silver provides sustained broad-spectrum bactericidal effects.	• 8 × 12 box = $$$ • 4 × 4 box = $$$ • 4 × 4 box = $$
Charcoal	CarboFlex (Convatec)	Absorbs small gas molecules and bacterial spores. Used as either primary or secondary dressings.	4 × 4 box = $$
Dakin's Solution 0.25% concentration	—	Broad-spectrum bactericidal effects, promotes dissolution of necrotic tissue. Requires twice-daily dressing changes.	1 16-oz bottle = $
Metronidazole	• 1% Flagyl spray • 5% Flagyl powder • Crushed tablets • 0.75% Flagyl gel	Bactericidal, effective against anaerobes.	• 100 mL = $ • 60 g = $ • 14 tablets = $ • 75% gel (1 tube, 45 g) = $$

Prices: $, <$100; $$, >$100; $$$, >$200.
Data from Refs.[38–40]; and *Prices from* Wound Care Shop. Available at: http://www.woundcareshop.com/. Accessed March 12, 2016.

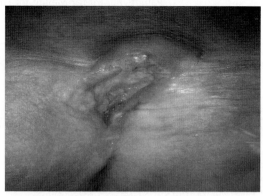

Fig. 5. Periwound moisture-associated dermatitis.

Table 2
Periwound skin management options

Skin Protectant	Description	Considerations	Examples
Liquid polymer acrylates	Liquid polymers that contain solvents that when they evaporate, form a protective film	Periwound maceration protection Preparation of skin attachment sites for drainage tubes, external catheters, surrounding ostomy sites, and adhesive dressings	Cavilon (3M) No-Sting Skin Prep (Smith & Nephew)
Dimethicone	Silicone-based oil	Modest maceration protection Good skin hydration Variable periwound skin irritant protection	Remedy Dimethicone Moisture Barrier (Medline)
Zinc oxide–based skin protectant	White powder mixed with a cream or ointment base	Periwound skin irritant protection Incontinence barrier Zinc offers poor skin hydration and does not avoid maceration Messy, difficult to remove Interfere with dressing adhesion and absorption	Medline Remedy Phytoplex Z-Guard Skin Protectant Paste (Medline) Critic-Aid Thick Moisture Barrier Skin Paste (Coloplast)
Petrolatum-based skin protectant	Blend of castor seed oil and hydrogenated castor oil	Periwound skin irritant and maceration protection Modest skin hydration Incontinence barrier Messy, difficult to remove Interfere with dressing adhesion and absorption	ConvaTec Sensi-Care Protective Barrier (ConvaTec) Medline Remedy Phytoplex Z-Guard Skin Protectant Paste (Medline)

Adapted from Colwell J, Ratliff C, Goldberg M, et al. MASD part 3: Peristomal moisture-associated dermatitis and periwound moisture-associated dermatitis, a consensus. J Wound Ostomy Continence Nurs 2011;38(5):541–53; with permission.

Treatment and prevention of pruritus caused by MASD starts with the selection of an appropriate absorbent dressing and cleansing of the wound bed. Periwound skin protection is the crucial next-step in preventing MASD with several product options available (**Table 2**).

To these authors knowledge, no study has specifically compared products used in periwound skin protection in patients with MFWs. A meta-analysis by Schuren and co-workers[46] in nonmalignant wounds found film barrier to be superior to placebo in four studies and no significant differences when compared with zinc oxide–based or petrolatum-based products.

Hospice formularies may already include petrolatum and zinc oxide–based skin barriers as part of their incontinence protocols. The authors recommend including a liquid-forming acrylate because it does not interfere with adherence of dressings or pouching appliances and is used to protect the skin from medical adhesive–related skin injury[47] and to prevent or treat MASD.[48]

Multiple considerations should be made when selecting a skin barrier including: location, allergies, and caregiver support. A liquid polymer acrylate for upper body, head, and facial wounds is appropriate because there is less mess, and no interference with adhesion of dressings. Consider a zinc oxide–based or petrolatum-based

---

Box 9
Bleeding etiologies in advanced cancer

- Malignant fungating wounds
  - Direct vessel invasion
  - Microvascular bleeding
    - Dressing selection/removal
    - Friable tissue: bioburden

- Thrombocytopenia
  - Chemotherapy
  - Paraneoplastic syndromes
  - Idiopathic thrombocytopenia purpura
  - Thrombotic thrombocytopenia
  - Invasion of tumor cells in bone marrow

- Cancers of the bone marrow
  - Multiple myeloma, leukemia, lymphoma

- Coagulopathy
  - Liver disease
    - Primary liver cancer
    - Metastatic liver cancer
  - Vitamin K deficiency

- Disseminated intravascular coagulation
  - Infection, malignancy, trauma

- High-dose chemotherapy
  - Cyclophosphamide

- Radiation (bone marrow production sites, such as ilia)

- Surgery

- Anticoagulation for deep venous thrombosis, pulmonary embolism, atrial fibrillation, stroke

Data from Camp-Sorrell D. Myelosuppresion. In: Itano J, Taoka K, editors. Core curriculum for oncology nursing. 4th edition. St Louis (MO): Elsevier Saunders; 2005. p. 264–7; and Gobel B. Metabolic emergencies. In: Itano J, Taoka K, editors. Core curriculum for oncology nursing. 4th edition. St Louis (MO): Elsevier Saunders; 2005. p. 383–8.

skin barrier for genital or groin wounds, especially in the presence of fecal or urinary incontinence.

The authors also recommend use of postsurgical bras (ie, Dale bras), Lycra, and Attends undergarments to secure dressings, normalize appearance, and reduce medical adhesive–related skin injury. Carrying an extra set of clothing in the event of strike through is also suggested.

PHYSICAL ASPECTS OF CARE: BLEEDING

Bleeding may range from superficial, isolated rupture of microvasculature in the wound bed to erosion of large vessels and hemorrhage. Disruption of blood vessels, either by direct tumor invasion or friable wound beds with excessive bioburden, was described by patients as "unpredictable."[4,19] The cause of bleeding in advanced cancer is usually multifactorial and may be thought of in terms of reversible and irreversible factors (**Box 9**).

Goals of care discussions surrounding bleeding are an integral part of advanced care planning for the hospice patient with an MFW because interventions may range from the benign (ie, direct pressure, vitamin K replacement, modification of topical antimicrobial therapy) to aggressive and/or invasive (ie, vascular interventions for hemorrhage, blood products, radiation). The discontinuation of anticoagulation for patients with atrial fibrillation, deep vein thrombosis, pulmonary embolism,

Table 3
Interventions for bleeding

Category of Bleeding	Interventions	Considerations
Prevention	Dressing selection and wound cleansing	Nonadherent dressings are recommended as a contact layer (silicone, foam, or petrolatum-based gauze) Gentle cleansing or irrigation Wet dressings before removal to loosen and prevent adherence to the wound bed
Minor bleeding (controllable at the bedside)	Direct pressure Silver nitrate Epinephrine soaks	Apply local pressure with clean gauze See **Fig. 6** Soak gauze with 1 mg of epinephrine and 1 mL of NS (1:1 ratio) applied for 10 minutes of direct pressure to promote local vasoconstriction[49]
	Calcium alginate	If using as a hemostatic agent, may embed itself in the wound and be difficult to extract
Major bleeding (requiring invasive or aggressive interventions)	Vascular interventions Radiation	Requires referral by an advanced practice clinician to vascular surgery or interventional radiology Requires referral by an advanced practice clinician to radiation oncology
Hemorrhage as a terminal event	Comfort measures	1. Dark towels should be readily available and used to contain and absorb blood loss 2. Sedate with a benzodiazepine and manage pain with an opioid 3. Cover with blankets because blood loss may cause hypothermia and chills

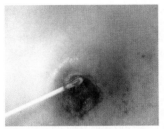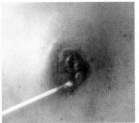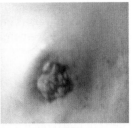

Fig. 6. Cauterization of bleeding abdominal malignant lesion with silver nitrate sticks. Note the stick is rolled over the bleeder causing a pearly gray appearance to the tissue. This may be repeated with each dressing change at bedside, is relatively inexpensive, and easy to learn. Assess for stinging or burning, and if uncomfortable consider alternatives.

or embolic stroke requires a discussion of risks versus benefits and must involve the advanced practice nurse or hospice medical director. If MFWs are in close proximity to large vessels (ie, femoral or carotid artery), the sensitive probing of patient wishes in the event of hemorrhage should be undertaken. This discussion

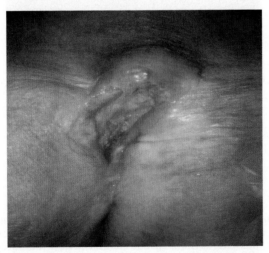

Fig. 7. Course of hospice care. Ms. C. **C:** On admission to IPU, screened positive for depression and anxiety, c/o painful MASD along the periwound/vaginal border, odor noted at the door of her room and exudates that stained her underwear and pants two to three times per day. C/o intermittent abdominal pain, not controlled with four to five doses of shortacting opioid. **A:** Friable, yellow-pink tissue with moderate yellow, foul exudates and circumferential periwound maceration and erythema. Odor noted at the door with dressing intact. **R:** Wound Care: Cleanse with warm soapy water via a peribottle, pat dry, 1% Flagyl spray to wound bed, petrolatum-based barrier periwound and ABD pads held in place by Attends undergarments. MASD resolved, odor and drainage were controlled within 3 days. Pain Management: Pain resolved with local care and a long-acting opioid and steroid with a short-acting opioid for breakthrough pain. The short-acting opioid was administered a half hour before wound care and again after completion if needed. Psychosocial: LCSW and Rabbi consulted for counseling, mirtazapine started, a shortacting benzodiazepine for anxiety as needed. **E:** IPU staff, patient, and her husband were educated in the wound care orders and protocol. The patient was able to participate in her own wound care but as her health and cognition failed, the staff assumed total responsibility until her death 2 weeks later.

should include comfort (sedation, pain management, temperature control, and family support) versus emergent transfer to a general inpatient level of care or acute care setting (ie, emergency room). **Table 3** highlights select interventions for bleeding.

SUMMARY

Lawton[19] observed that certain nursing interventions and adequate symptom management could once again bind the body, alleviating suffering and palliating the patient and family's psychological distress. Through the use of a systematic, holistic approach (PALCARE) guided by a palliative wound care specialist, the hospice team was able to address the complex physical, psychosocial, and spiritual needs of Ms. C and Ms. A (**Figs. 7** and **8**).

This article highlights the need for an interdisciplinary approach to palliative wound care guided by specialist-level expertise. A holistic approach to caring for patients with MFWs or any wounds at end-of-life includes considering PALCARE.

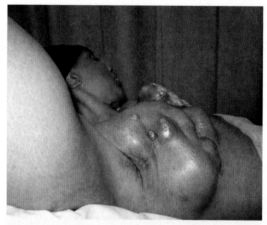

Fig. 8. Course of hospice care. Ms. A. **C**: On admission to IPU, screened negative for depression and anxiety, c/o painful MASD circumferentially periwound and constant right chest wall aching with intermittent burning, not controlled with short-acting opioids every 4 hours. Odor was noted down the hall and exudates stained her clothes with dressing changes every 2 to 3 hours. **A**: Left chest wall/sternal MFW 25 cm x17 cm x 5 cm (depth),cauliflower appearance with pockets of friable, bleeding tissue, large amount of creamy, yellow, foul exudate with circumferential periwound maceration and erythema. Odor was noted as one walked onto the unit. Right arm lymphedema with extensive tumor burden right chest wall. **R**: Wound Care: 7 days of quarterstrength Dakins packing every 12 hours, then cleanse and gently irrigate with warm soapy water via a peribottle, pat/air dry, silver nitrate cauterization PRN, 5% Flagyl powder to wound bed, nonadherent petrolatum-gauze, liquid polymer acrylate periwound, and ABD pads held in place by a Dale bra. Dressings started every 12 hours for 5 days then daily. MASD resolved, odor and drainage were controlled within 7 days. For fevers and chills, a 5- day course of oral Flagyl was completed. Pain Management: Pain was controlled with a long-acting opioid, a steroid and a short-acting opioid for breakthrough pain. The short-acting opioid was administered a half hour before wound care and again after completion if needed. Psychosocial: LCSW consulted for counseling and discharge planning. **E**: The IPU staff and patient were educated in the wound care orders/ protocol. The patient was able to independently perform her own wound care, including silver nitrate cauterization and was transferred home 2.5 weeks later.

In addition to a methodical approach to care, this article also makes clear the need for rigorous interventional research in palliative wound, ostomy, and continence care. Evidence-based nursing is the key to providing high-quality palliative care and alleviating the multidimensional suffering experienced by patients and families at end-of-life.

REFERENCES

1. Naylor W. Malignant wounds, aetiology and principles of management. Nurs Stand 2002;16:45–53.
2. Grocott P, Gethin G, Probst S. Malignant wound management in advanced illness: new insights. Curr Opin Support Palliat Care 2013;7:101–5.
3. Lo S, Hu W, Hayter M, et al. Experiences of living with a malignant fungating wound: a qualitative study. J Clin Nurs 2008;17(20):2699–708.
4. Probst S, Arber A, Faithfull S. Coping with an ulcerative breast carcinoma; an interpretive phenomenological study. J Wound Care 2013;22(7):352–60.
5. Adderley U, Smith R. Topical agents and dressing for fungating wounds. Cochrane Database Syst Rev 2007;(2):CD003948.
6. Lund-Nielsen B, Midtgaard J, Rorth M, et al. An avalanche of ignoring: a qualitative study of health care avoidance in women with malignant breast cancer wounds. Cancer Nurs 2011;34(4):277–85.
7. Seamen S, Bates-Jensen B. Skin disorders; malignant wounds, fistulas, and stomas. In: Ferrell B, Coyle N, Paice J, editors. Oxford textbook of palliative nursing. 4th edition. New York: Oxford University Press; 2015. p. 325–40.
8. Woo K, Sibbald G. Local wound care for malignant and palliative wounds. Adv Skin Wound Care 2010;23:417–28.
9. Grocott P. The palliative management of fungating malignant wounds. J Wound Care 1995;4(5):240–2.
10. Mortimer P. Skin problems in palliative care: medical aspects. In: Doyle D, Hanks G, Macdonald N, editors. Oxford textbook of palliative medicine. 3rd edition. Oxford: Oxford Medical Publications; 1993. p. 384–95.
11. O'Brien C. Malignant wounds: managing odor. Can Fam Physician 2012;58: 272–3.
12. Dolbeault S, Flahault C, Baffie A, et al. Psychological profile of patients with neglected malignant wounds: a qualitative exploratory study. J Wound Care 2010;19(12):513–21.
13. Gibson S, Green J. Review of patient's experiences with fungating wounds and associated quality of life. J Wound Care 2013;22(5):265–75.
14. Grocott P, Browne N, Cowley S. Quality of life: assessing the impact and benefits of care to patients with fungating wounds. Wounds 2005;17(1):8–15.
15. Lo S, Hayter M, Hu W, et al. Symptom burden and quality of life in patients with malignant fungating wounds. J Adv Nurs 2012;68:1312–21.
16. WOCN. News and press: products and publications. 2010. Available at: http://www. wocn.org/news/67111/Purchase-a-Copy-of-the-WOC-Nursing-Scope–Standards-of-Practice.htm. Accessed February 3, 2016.
17. WOCN. Scope and standards of practice. Mt Laurel (NJ): WOCN; 2010.
18. NINR. NINR research: investing in the future. 2015. Available at: http://www.nih. gov/about/almanac/organization/NINR.htm. Accessed February 3, 2016.
19. Lawton J. Contemporary hospice care: the sequestration of the unbounded body and "dirty dying". Sociol Health Illn 1998;20(2):121–43.

20. Probst S, Arber A, Faithfull S. Malignant fungating wounds: the meaning of living in an unbounded body. Eur J Oncol Nurs 2013;17:38–45.

21. Piggin C, Jones V. Malignant fungating wounds: an analysis of the lived experience. J Wound Care 2009;18(2):57–64.

22. Young CV. The effects of malodorous fungating malignant wounds on body image and quality of life. J Wound Care 2005;14(8):359–62.

23. Lund-Nielsen B, Adamsen L, Kolmos H, et al. The effect of honey-coated bandages compared with silver-coated bandages on treatment of malignant wounds-a randomized study. Wound Repair Regen 2011;19:664–70.

24. Bredin M. Mastectomy, body image and therapeutic massage: a qualitative study of women's experience. J Adv Nurs 1999;29(5):1113–20.

25. Fenton S. Reflections on lymphoedema, fungating wounds and the power of touch in the last weeks of life. Int J Palliat Nurs 2011;17(2):60–6.

26. Hawthorn M. Caring for a patient with a fungating malignant lesion in a hospice setting: reflecting on practice. Int J Palliat Nurs 2010;16(2):70–6.

27. Harmer V. Breast cancer part 3: advanced cancer and psychological implications. Br J Nurs 2008;17(17):1088–98.

28. Seamen S. Management of malignant fungating wounds in advanced cancer. Semin Oncol Nurs 2006;22(3):185–93.

29. Alexander SJ. An intense and unforgettable experience: the lived experience of malignant wounds from the perspectives of patients, caregivers, and nurses. Int Wound J 2010;7(6):456–65.

30. The FICA Spiritual History Tool. George Washington University School of Medicine & Health Sciences website. Available at: https://smhs.gwu.edu/gwish/clinical/fica. Accessed February 13, 2016.

31. Naylor W. Assessment and management of pain in fungating wounds. Br J Nurs 2001;10(22):S33–52.

32. Woo K, Sibbald G, Fogh K, et al. Assessment and management of persistent (chronic) and total wound pain. Int Wound J 2008;5(2):205–15.

33. Probst S. Evidence-based management of fungating wounds. Wounds (Palliative Wound Care Supplement). 2010.

34. Price P, Fogh K, Glynn C, et al. Managing painful chronic wounds: the wound pain management model. Int Wound J 2007;4(Suppl 1):4–15.

35. Mehta A, Chan L. Understanding of the concept of "total pain". J Hosp Palliat Nurs 2008;10(1):26–32.

36. Walsh A, Bradley M, Cavallito K. Management of fungating tumors and pressure ulcers in a patient with stage IV cutaneous malignant melanoma. J Hosp Palliat Nurs 2014;16(4):208–14.

37. Kalemikerakis J. Comparison of foam dressings with silver versus foam dressings without silver in the care of malodorous malignant fungating wounds. J BUON 2012;17(3):560–4.

38. Hampton S. Malodorous fungating wounds: how dressings alleviate symptoms. Br J Community Nurs 2008;13:S31–8.

39. Smith & Nephew. Allevyn Adhesive. Available at: http://www.smith-nephew.com/key-products/advanced-woundmanagement/allevyn/allevyn-adhesive/. Accessed March 12, 2016.

40. Dermasciences. Algicell Ag Education. Available at: http://www.dermasciences.com/algicell-education. Accessed March 12, 2016.

41. Cutting KF, White RJ. Avoidance and management of periwound maceration of the skin. Prof Nurse 2002;18(1):33, 35–6.

42. Cutting KF, White RJ. Maceration of the skin and wound bed: its nature and causes. J Wound Care 2002;11(7):275–8.
43. Van Rijswijk L, Catanzaro J. Wound assessment and documentation. In: Krasner D, Rodeheaver G, Sibbald R, editors. Chronic wound care: a clinical source book for health care professionals. 4th edition. Malvern (PA): HMP Communications; 2007. p. 113–26.
44. Gray M, Weir D. Prevention and treatment of moisture-associated skin damage (maceration) in the periwound skin. J Wound Ostomy Continence Nurs 2007; 34:153–7.
45. Tamai N, Akase T, Minematsu T, et al. Association between components of exudates and periwound moisture-associated dermatitis in breast cancer patients with malignant fungating wounds. Biol Res Nurs 2016;18(2):199–206.
46. Schuren J, Becker A, Sibbald RA. Liquid film-forming acrylate for peri-wound protection: a systematic review and meta-analysis (3M Cavilon no-sting barrier film). Int Wound J 2005;2:230–8.
47. McNichol L, Lund C, Rosen T, et al. Medical adhesives and patient safety: state of the science: consensus statements for the assessment, prevention, and treatment of adhesive-related skin injuries. J Wound Ostomy Continence Nurs 2013; 40(4):367–80.
48. Colwell J, Ratliff C, Goldberg M, et al. MASD part 3: peristomal moisture-associated dermatitis and periwound moisture-associated dermatitis, a consensus. J Wound Ostomy Continence Nurs 2011;38(5):541–53.
49. Hulme B, Wilcox S. Guidelines on management of bleeding in palliative care patients with Cancer. 2008. Available at: www.palliativedrugs.com/download/090331_Final_bleeding_guideline.pdf. Accessed February 25, 2016.

Index

Note: Page numbers of article titles are in **boldface** type.

A

Adult patients, animal-assisted care in palliative care for, 384–385
    noncommunicative, pain assessment in palliative care for, **397–431**
Advance care planning, of LGBTQ patients, 503–504
Animal-assisted care, in pediatric palliative care, **381–395**
        in adults, 384–385
        background, 382–383
        in children, 385–389
        current and future research, 390–391
        definition of, 384
        limitations, 388–389
        practice implications, 389–390
        types of, 383–384
Annointing with oil, at end of life, 480

B

Baptism, at end of life, 479, 487
        supplies needed for, 487
Behavioral Pain Scales, use in noncommunicative adult palliative care patients, 400, 409
Bisexuals. *See* LGBTQ patients.
Bleeding, in palliative care for malignant fungating wounds, 525–527

C

Ceremonies, honoring, at end of life, 477–478
Checklist of Nonverbal Pain Indicators, for noncommunicative adult palliative care patients, 409, 418
Children. *See* Pediatric palliative care.
Chronic care, Medicare reimbursement for, 375
Communication skills, for integrating palliative care into primary care, 371–372
Community resources, for integrating palliative care into primary care, 372–373
Complementary and alternative medicine, role in palliative wound care for malignant fungating wounds, 519
Continence. *See* Wound care, palliative.
Critical Care Pain Observation Tool, use in noncommunicative adult palliative care patients, 418–419
Critical care setting, end-of-life rituals in, 474–475

D

Death, collective responses to, 480–481
Deathbed phenomena, **489–500**

Nurs Clin N Am 51 (2016) 533–544
http://dx.doi.org/10.1016/S0029-6465(16)30046-9
0029-6465/16/$ – see front matter

Moving?

Make sure your subscription moves with you!

To notify us of your new address, find your **Clinics Account Number** (located on your mailing label above your name), and contact customer service at:

Email: journalscustomerservice-usa@elsevier.com

800-654-2452 (subscribers in the U.S. & Canada)
314-447-8871 (subscribers outside of the U.S. & Canada)

Fax number: 314-447-8029

Elsevier Health Sciences Division
Subscription Customer Service
3251 Riverport Lane
Maryland Heights, MO 63043

ELSEVIER